Understanding Chronic Fatigue Syndrome

Understanding Chronic Fatigue Syndrome

AN EMPIRICAL GUIDE TO ASSESSMENT AND TREATMENT

FRED FRIEDBERG

LEONARD A. JASON

AMERICAN PSYCHOLOGICAL ASSOCIATION
WASHINGTON, DC

Published by
American Psychological Association
750 First Street, NE
Washington, DC 20002

Copies may be ordered from
APA Order Department
P.O. Box 92984
Washington, DC 20090-2984

In the United Kingdom, Europe, Africa, and the Middle East, copies may be ordered from
American Psychological Association
3 Henrietta Street
Covent Garden
London WC2E 8LU
England

Typeset in Meridien by Harlowe Typography, Cottage City, MD

Printer: Braun-Brumfield, Inc., Ann Arbor, MI
Jacket designer: Berg Design, Albany, NY
Jacket illustrator: Jim Sande, Albany, NY
Technical/production editor: Valerie Montenegro

Library of Congress Cataloging-in-Publication Data
Friedberg, Fred.
    Understanding chronic fatigue syndrome : an empirical guide to
  assessment and treatment / Fred Friedberg and Leonard A. Jason. —
  1st ed.
        p.   cm.
    Includes bibliographical references and index.
    ISBN 1-55798-511-1 (cloth : acid-free paper)
    1. Chronic fatigue syndrome.   I. Jason, Leonard.   II. Title.
    [DNLM: 1. Fatigue Syndrome, Chronic—diagnosis.   2.   Fatigue
  Syndrome, Chronic—therapy.   WB 146 F899u 1998]
  RB150.F37F753   1998
  616'.0478—dc21
  for Library of Congress   98-21293
                                                                 CIP

British Library Cataloguing-in-Publication Data
A CIP record is available from the British Library.

Printed in the United States of America
First edition

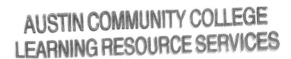

Contents

APPENDIXES

Foreword
Unrecognized Illness:
Who Suffers? What Can Be Done?

When individuals become ill and are subjected to multiple tests by physicians, including blood chemistry analyses, CAT scans, and MRIs, they want to have a medical answer to their suffering. Many of my chronic fatigue syndrome (CFS) patients say they would rather have cancer than not know what was making them feel like they were dying. With cancer there is a known pathophysiology, even if the cure (when available) may be painful.

Who Suffers?

PATIENTS

Individuals who have complaints about constant weakness, fatigue, and sore throats want to be taken seriously. They may look fine and normal but they describe themselves as feeling like "death warmed over." Of great concern to many is a pronounced cognitive slippage involving loss of memory and difficulties with sustained attention. Almost all of these individuals attribute their symptoms to a physical cause and seek a medical solution.

In the history of medicine, the failure to find an "organic basis" to a problem typically leads to the conclusion, "It must be in the patient's head." This attitude is the source of much frustration for patients who are beset with an endless array of varying symptoms that rob them of the predictability of daily life. Now they find themselves in the awkward position of having to justify that they indeed have a legitimate problem.

PARTNERS

The patient is not the only frustrated individual. Relationships with partners and significant others suffer as well. Individuals with CFS are often asked if they feel "up to" participating in activities. Partners often assume that they are "too wiped out" and may limit invitations with other people. Thus, partners are also involuntary prisoners to this disorder, not knowing what to do to help or what not to do. This uncertainty may hinder the recovery of their loved one. Sometimes the partner's efforts are appreciated, but these efforts may also be seen as overprotective or patronizing.

PHYSICIANS

In addition, society punishes the physician who is supposed to be a healer but who is denied the ability to administer effective treatment or the "magic pill," as we might wish. So the National Institutes of Health, Institute of Allergy and Infectious Diseases admits in its treatise for the physician that "despite multidisciplinary investigations into the cause of CFS, its etiology remains unknown."[1] Given such limited knowledge, they recommend a "supportive program of patient management—including symptom-based treatment, education about the disease, and regular follow-up visits to rule out alternative diagnoses" (p. 3).

The healer's limited assignment, to educate patients about the disease and seek out alternative diagnoses, again belies a sense of helplessness regarding this entity known as Chronic Fatigue Syndrome.

EMPLOYERS AND SOCIETY

Employers may also lose a valuable resource, in that work environments usually do not allow flexibility to individuals who can work only when energy levels permit. Thus, many persons who develop CFS become frustrated and demoralized in their attempts to maintain employment at premorbid levels and may have little choice but to leave their jobs and seek disability benefits.

---

[1]From *What Physicians Know About Chronic Fatigue Syndrome* (p. 3) by National Institute of Allergy and Infectious Diseases, 1997, Washington, DC: U.S. Government Printing Office.

The tax on society is also great. In addition to paying disability compensation, health care costs escalate because of physician shopping for a more definitive diagnosis or the elusive treatment that might work. Society also loses many previously able-bodied individuals who are excluded from the workplace. The cognitive loss of self-esteem that accompanies such displacement often results in concurrent depression in individuals with CFS.

Making Sense of This Illness

WHY WOMEN MAY PRESENT MORE FREQUENTLY THAN MEN

Nowhere is the issue of women suffering societal biases more pertinent than in the interface between medical and psychological problems. Women are three times more likely than men to receive the diagnosis of CFS. Gender-related differences are varied, with women showing more tender lymph nodes, fibromyalgia, and lower physical functioning; in contrast, men show more pharyngeal inflammation and a higher lifetime prevalence of alcohol misuse.

Historically, women have had bad public relations about their medical complaints. Their depiction as hysterical females, with lack of real symptoms has endured since earliest times.[2] Unfortunately, we are once again in the Dark Ages as women face the cultural debate over CFS, fact or fiction.

Women may be more likely than men to receive a diagnosis of CFS. Why? Because women are more verbally expressive regarding their emotions, they often reach diagnostic criteria for psychiatric as well as medical disorders when concurrent labels are applied. Thus, we see a threefold ratio of women to men even in areas where community data suggests equal prevalence.

EPIDEMICS AND CFS

CFS has been identified in both sporadic and clustered cases. In some instances, localized epidemics have occurred. What constitutes an epidemic? Most people think of a calamitous occurrence of deadly infectious disease such as the Black Death. Medical science defines

---

[2]*From Paralysis to Fatigue* by E. Shorter, 1991, New York: Macmillan.

epidemic as a disease or damaging health event with an unusually strong adverse effect on the health of the population. It is defined in terms of geography, and the personal characteristics of those who contract the disease or experience the adverse health event.

Over the past several decades, CFS and CFS-like illnesses have sometimes appeared as isolated epidemics, often affecting schools, hospitals, or other institutions where there is close contact among members. Medical investigators surmised that these disease outbreaks must have been precipitated by an infectious agent. Many research dollars were spent to investigate possible viral or immune-related problems. Unfortunately, the heterogeneity of this population of sufferers has obscured the identification of a consistent marker for the disease. But well-designed prevalence studies can inform us of the magnitude of both the sporadic and the clustered outbreaks of CFS. CFS epidemiologist and coauthor Leonard Jason provides an up-to-date overview of prevalence studies and compares their findings to popular CFS stereotypes (e.g., yuppie flu).

DISEASE VERSUS ILLNESS

The distinction between disease and illness is also an important consideration in CFS. *Disease* refers to an entity that physicians diagnose and treat, whereas *illness* refers to the experience of disease, including the feelings relating to changes in bodily states and the consequences of having to bear that ailment. Because people with CFS feel ill, they understandably assume that they have a disease. They may suffer symptoms for some time before seeking medical advice. However, if medical evaluation reveals no objective markers of disease, this does not banish their claim to "feel ill."

Given patients' experiences of medical rejection, their concerns and fears may escalate to anger, which may in turn further affect their functioning and compromise their immune systems. Although medical science has not yet pinpointed any specific immune deficiencies, considerable physiologic variability has been found in the sympathetic and parasympathetic nervous systems of individuals with CFS. This variability may in part reflect a hypersensitivity to stress that may be an inherent property of CFS and perhaps a causal factor as well.

THE "SICK ROLE" AND CFS

Parsons and Fox construe illness and health as social dimensions.[3] "Falling ill" involves the individual assuming a "sick role." Doctors are

---

[3]"Illness, Therapy, and the Modern Urban American Family" by T. Parsons and R. Fox, 1952, *Journal of Social Issues, 8,* 31–44.

then sought to return people to their normal physical and social lives. Yet doctors deem some groups of sufferers as more justified in their "sick role" than others. So with an illness that professionals themselves have failed to recognize and treat, it is likely that the CFS sufferer is not given the recognition awarded others who have illnesses that are verified by a disease process and legitimized by the physician. Thus, in desperation, many CFS patients may dramatize their situation in order that others may grasp their experience and credit them with having a genuine illness.[4]

What Is the Best Treatment?

In the absence of effective medical treatments or cure, the ability to adjust psychologically to the illness is an important element of any intervention. The treatments recommended in this book combine cognitive restructuring, coping skills training, stress management, and behavior modification. Skillful application of these interventions can constructively influence the coping abilities and activity levels of the patient. Significantly, these treatments can also quell the tide of trauma arising from the disabling realities of CFS. In contrast to well-publicized graded activity treatments, author Fred Friedberg, an experienced CFS clinician and researcher, believes that patients need to pace their activity in order to conserve energy and avoid overexertion and relapse.

Enlarging on this energy conserving strategy, coauthor and research psychologist Leonard Jason uses the envelope theory as the basis of a new treatment.[5] Envelope theory provides a testable hypothesis that predicts that if the patient's perceived energy and expended energy are properly balanced, people with CFS can avoid relapse while increasing their tolerance to activity. Thus, the appropriate level of activity needs to be assessed person by person. Although the authors recognize the need for researchers to hone in on clinically important subgroups of patients who experience this illness, they also applaud in vivo approaches that capture the ebb and flow of symptoms, activity, and stress levels for each individual with the illness.

---

[4]*The Presentation of Self in Everyday Life* by E. Goffman, 1971, Harmondswoth, England: Penguin.

[5]*Recovering From Chronic Fatigue Syndrome* by W. Collinge, 1993, New York: The Body Press/Perigee.

We have in this refreshing volume a first real attempt to combine science and therapy to present the state of the art in the assessment and treatment of CFS.

I highly recommend this sophisticated book to all professionals working in the field, be they clinicians or researchers. The material presented will both enlighten and challenge, as well as provide the most constructive approach to dealing with the symptoms and frustrations of these sufferers.

BARBARA G. MELAMED, PhD

Preface

When chronic fatigue syndrome (CFS) was first defined and publicly recognized in the late 1980s, there was a media frenzy on the subject generated by the mystery of a poorly understood illness and the controversy about its origins. Was it a form of depression, as some suggested, or perhaps an imaginary illness, created by greedy yuppies who became sick in protest because they couldn't have it all? Or was it a form of malingering to gain sympathy and attention? Given this widespread skepticism in combination with the absence of medical findings, CFS patients had to try to convince their doctors that they were suffering from a very real and disabling illness.

Although the media frenzy has died down, the illness has not gone away. Actually, recent prevalence studies suggest that this debilitating condition is far more common than was previously thought. However, the government's response to the illness has been slow, inconsistent, and, we believe, inadequate. By contrast, another contemporary serious illness, AIDS, has captured considerably more attention from public health officials and scientists. Perhaps this is understandable, given the number of people who have died of this lethal disease, as well as the number of high-profile individuals who have been infected with HIV. Thousands of scientists have worked in the area of HIV/AIDS research, and many government programs have been developed for those with this disease. Regrettably, medical research scientists and funding agencies expressed a very different reaction for those suffering from CFS.

Skepticism about the illness was widespread and research support was almost nonexistent.

When we began conducting research on CFS in the early 1990s, the first published reports of high rates of psychiatric comorbidity allowed many health professions to surmise that CFS was a psychiatric illness, perhaps a form of depression with somatic symptoms. But CFS patients' frequent complaints of flu-like symptoms led some research groups to investigate the possibility that a persistent viral illness or an immune defect caused the illness. However, when laboratory studies revealed no consistent viral or immunological abnormality in CFS samples, many more health care professionals concluded that this disorder was a psychiatric illness.

Although we recognize that medical markers have not yet been found, the unusual symptomatic picture of CFS leads us to believe that the illness cannot be primarily explained as a psychiatric condition. Extremely successful people have had their lives shattered after developing CFS, and it appears that these individuals had little to gain by adopting a sick role, as some theorists have suggested. For other fatiguing illnesses, like multiple sclerosis and Lyme disease, biological markers were ultimately identified after years of research. Before such markers were found, many health professionals also viewed these debilitating conditions as psychiatric disorders. We believe that the pathophysiological mechanisms underlying CFS will eventually be discovered. Given that CFS has both biologic and psychiatric aspects, psychologists can play a key role in developing research strategies to better understand this syndrome.

Over the past decade and a half, the field of CFS has generated a research literature on proposed causation, clinical course, epidemiology, medical and psychological assessment, and approaches to clinical intervention. In this book, we summarize the research and clinical work that has been done, particularly since 1990, in order to provide an updated and comprehensive analysis of the illness. During this recent period, a new case definition has been proposed, a second generation of more valid epidemiological studies has been conducted, more sophisticated assessment methods have been evaluated, and more rigorous treatment studies have been published.

Significantly, psychologists and other mental health professionals around the world have joined medical research teams to conduct and publish research in the area of CFS. Because these publications are found primarily in medical journals, the mental health professional may be less familiar with clinical and scientific work relevant to CFS. Yet psychotherapists have become increasingly aware of individuals with CFS as they present themselves for help in coping with their illness. However, mental health clinicians have not had a professional reference volume to help them understand, assess, and treat this puzzling condition. The material in this book will help mental health professionals gain the resources and information they need to better serve those with CFS. For psychological and medical research scientists, this volume provides a review and synthesis of psychological and biological data on CFS. It also offers a detailed presentation of the self-report fatigue scales and psychometric instruments that are important for baseline and follow-up evaluations.

For the hundreds of thousands of people with CFS, few professionals are available who have both the knowledge and the sensitivity to care for these patients. Our hope is that this book will (a) stimulate practicing psychologists and other mental health professionals to develop more sensitive assessment and treatment strategies and (b) assist CFS scientists in developing more theoretically rigorous and valid research methodologies.

Acknowledgments

The authors are deeply appreciative of many colleagues who have helped shape the ideas in this book, including Pat Fennell, Judy Richman, Karen Jordan, Doreen Salina, Andy and Sigita Plioplys, David Lipkin, Morris Papernik, Wendell Richmond, Bill McReadie, Fred Rademaker, Joseph Ferrari, Warren Tryon, Jackie Golding, Stephen Goldston, and Barbara Pino.

We are also most appreciative of our friends who have done so much to educate us about the needs of those with CFS. They include Darryl Isenberg, Carol Howard, Jim LeRoy, Sarah Labelle, Harriet Melrose, Marty Greenberg, Dvorah Budnick, Joyce Goodlatte, Nicki Savich, Laura Distelheim, Susan Rosenthal, Ruth Robins, Diane Allene, Beth Ferris, Ken Lipman, Lisa Schicht, Nancy Flynn, and Mona Campbell. We are also deeply indebted to our many students who have patiently taught us so much, including Renee Taylor, Lynne Wagner, Stephanie Taylor, Sharon Johnson, Jennifer Shlaes, Erin Frankenberry, Caroline King, Dana Landis, Susan Torres, Trina Haney, Jennifer Camacho, Peter Bishop, Amy Kolak, Tanya Pernell, Susan Slavich, Cheryl Stenzel, Michael Ropacki, John Holden, Genevieve Fitzgibbon, Karen Danner, and Dan Cantillon.

Concerning the editorial staff at the American Psychological Association, including Andrea Phillippi and Mary Lynn Skutley, we greatly appreciate their support and encouragement.

Finally, we wish to thank our families who have been a continual source of inspiration as we wrote this book.

OVERVIEW

History, Definition, and Prevalence

Because chronic fatigue syndrome (CFS) patients vary considerably in their clinical presentations and often report a number of perplexing medical and psychiatric symptoms, it is useful to look at case studies to better appreciate the nature of the symptom complex. Consider the following case vignettes:

> When Denise became pregnant for the first time at age 38, she and her husband were elated. However, during her second trimester, she began to experience generalized muscle aches and joint pain, memory problems, continuous fatigue, rashes, and one-sided headaches. These debilitating symptoms persisted after the birth of her twins. Her family doctor, finding no definitive medical explanation or treatment for her symptoms, diagnosed CFS and attributed the illness to chronic antibiotic use over many years for chronic vaginal infections. Denise was extremely frustrated by her condition and the resulting inability to return to her job as a police officer.
>
> After 21 months of persistent illness, she attended five sessions of coping skills and stress reduction therapy. Initially, she recognized that her bouts of (unfounded) worry about having a life-threatening illness, such as AIDS, were exacerbating her physical symptoms of sore throat and generalized muscle aches. Worry-reducing coping statements helped to ease these fears. By charting her symptoms and activity, she also learned that her chronic muscle aches were due in part to daily 15-minute walks. Such "exercise intolerance" is a key symptom of CFS. As she learned to pace her activity, the muscle aches

lessened. In addition, relaxation exercises helped to ease her sleeping difficulties and reduced the daily stress of caring for two infants. Her increased ability to control these symptoms made her feel more hopeful about further improvements and lessened the marital strains caused by the illness.

* * *

Bill had enjoyed excellent health all his life until 18 months ago, when, at age 58, he began experiencing severe headaches followed by overwhelming fatigue, joint pains, tender lymph glands, and poor sleep. A complete medical examination, including an MRI of the brain, yielded normal results. His physician, by excluding other potential explanations for these symptoms, diagnosed CFS. Bill was forced to give up his successful private law practice due to fatigue-related disability. His marriage of 2 years was strained because of his physical limitations, and he lost his sexual desire. Most disturbing to him were the cognitive problems of mental confusion, poor attention, and frequent forgetfulness. These cognitive difficulties prevented him from working as little as 2 hours a day.

Given the absence of effective medical treatment for CFS, he attended 15 coping skills and stress management sessions. Through the course of therapy, he began to recognize that his wife's unwillingness to assume a more traditional caretaker role with him was a source of his resentment, anger flare-ups, personal guilt, and worry about a second marital failure. In retrospect, he believed that this persistent and intense emotional distress may have contributed to the development of CFS. Yet his illness did not produce a "secondary gain" of increased attention from his wife. Instead, she was frustrated by his limitations and did not curtail any of her numerous personal activities. Furthermore, he lost friends as a result of his inability to maintain social and recreational activities.

The coping skills and cognitive restructuring intervention focused on (a) stress reduction techniques for persistent worry and physical tension, (b) daily activity pacing for CFS symptom management, and (c) identification and reevaluation of his views about potential marital partners. Bill made progress in all these areas, including improvements in the debilitating mental fogginess. This newfound control over his cognitive symptoms provided him with hope that he could learn to cope better with the illness. Over a 12-month period of personal rehabilitation, his illness gradually improved, although he remained too symptomatic to resume full-time work. Fortunately, his private disability insurance provided the financial support he needed during this slow recovery process.

* * *

Beth's fatiguing illness began 7 years ago. She experienced moderate but manageable levels of flu-like fatigue that lasted for several weeks and alternated with periods of high energy and hyperactivity. Over the past 2 years, she developed full-blown

CFS (diagnosed by her physician) with symptoms of severe flu-like headaches, crushing exhaustion, joint pains, concentration difficulty, and postexertional symptom flare-ups. In addition, she reported a number of other symptoms often associated with CFS, including panic attacks, dizzy spells, blurred vision, and light sensitivity. At 31, Beth had become unable to work and remained home. Fortunately, her husband provided physical and emotional support.

The apparent trigger for her CFS was a job transfer to a high-pressure school administrator position that required 60-hour work weeks. The work-related stress led to sleep disturbances, poor appetite, and increasing exhaustion states. At the same time, Beth had attempted to maintain her high-powered lifestyle of daily exercise, social commitments, and volunteer activities.

Over a 12-month period of coping skills and stress reduction therapy, Beth recognized that (a) her symptoms were highly stress-sensitive; (b) her failure to meet her perfectionist self-demands for accomplishment were inducing anxiety, guilt, and depressed mood; and (c) her strong approval needs generated persistent anxiety and CFS symptom exacerbations. As Beth learned to alleviate stress with relaxation techniques and to rethink her self-demands with cognitive coping skills, her symptom control improved substantially. Over a 2-year period, she recovered 70 to 80% of her premorbid functioning, although she remained susceptible to stress-induced setbacks that could persist for several weeks. A course of sertraline (Zoloft) was also helpful for managing symptoms of anxiety and depression.

The preceding case vignettes illustrate the wide range of symptoms and functional limitations found among these patients. It should be noted that, although many people with CFS experience improvements over time, complete recovery is rare. Also, a substantial minority of patients worsen over time. This is in contrast to primary depression and anxiety disorders that may go into extended periods of remission with or without clinical treatment. CFS is most likely caused by a complex set of interactive precipitating and maintaining conditions. An understanding of this disease requires an appreciation of diverse regions of psychology and other disciplines, such as psychoneuroimmunology. Indeed, it demands an understanding of the interrelationships between both psychological and biological—mind *and* body—variables.

This book aims to synthesize these variables in light of theory, data, and practice. This integration is accomplished both in chapters specifically devoted to assessment procedures for CFS and in chapters that describe various treatment models, such as cognitive–behavioral intervention, and medical and alternative therapies. This introductory chapter offers a broad overview of the history of this enigmatic illness and summarizes research findings on the demographics, prevalence, and prognosis for CFS. The chapter concludes with a discussion of the general scope and organization of the book.

A Brief History

Serious, disabling chronic fatigue is not a new, late twentieth-century kind of malaise. The history dates back at least 100 years, and with that history unfolds a complex, contradictory, and often controversial picture of a puzzling illness. We will briefly trace its historical roots, noting how medical, psychological, and sociocultural models of unexplained fatiguing illness have evolved. These earlier models foreshadow the current conflicts among theoreticians, researchers, and clinicians about the nature of CFS. These controversies will be explored in the remainder of the book.

THE RISE AND FALL OF NEURASTHENIA

Wessely (1990) suggested that myalgic encephalomyelitis (the term used for CFS in Great Britain) had its origins in the last century with the condition known as neurasthenia. George Beard, an American neurologist, was responsible for publicizing the disease, beginning in 1869 (Beard, 1869). He viewed this disabling condition as an entirely organic illness of profound fatigability of the body and mind. By the late 1800s, neurasthenia was one of the most frequently diagnosed illnesses. Weir Mitchell, a fellow neurologist, proposed a "rest cure" that was later offered by private sanatoria. The rest cure prescription, in its extreme form, dictated total bedrest punctuated only by bathroom breaks. Patients were not permitted to read, write, think too hard, or even brush their teeth.

Charlotte Perkins Gilman's (1993) famous short story, *The Yellow Wallpaper,* placed the rest cure in the cultural context of the late nineteenth century. The heroine of this tale was ordered to rest in an isolated room and was denied all visitors and reading materials. The story was a metaphor for the lives of middle-class women trapped in other people's expectations; the patient's Victorian physicians told her to rest until she wanted to pursue only "natural" womanly activities rather than the "unwomanly" intellectual activities that she craved. She eventually went mad, the only way she could become "free." An excellent discussion of the rest treatment approach for neurasthenia may be found in Ehrenreich and English's (1989) book, *For Her Own Good: 150 Years of Experts' Advice to Women.*

By World War I, the diagnosis of neurasthenia had almost disappeared. According to Wessely (1990), this change occurred as increasing medical skepticism and psychiatric sophistication led to the view that neurasthenia was a psychiatric rather than a neurological condition. In addition, the illness was increasingly perceived as an affliction of the lower social classes. It is not clear what influences led to these changing perceptions. Perhaps the upper classes rejected illnesses that had psychiatric implications, whereas those with fewer resources and limited access to needed care might have been more likely to be stigmatized with psychiatric labels. The diagnosis of neurasthenia was eventually discredited and became shameful for patients to confess.

UNEXPLAINED FATIGUING ILLNESS: WWI TO THE 1980s

The illness now known as CFS was less reported from WWI to the early 1980s. One or more of the following possibilities may have accounted for this decline: (a) the illness was, in fact, less prevalent; (b) physicians were less likely to diagnose it; (c) patients were less inclined to bring their complaints to physicians, who tended to perceive those complaints in psychiatric terms. It is unclear which one or combination of the three possible explanations account for the decrease in CFS reporting. However, we believe that explanations (b) and (c) are more plausible. In an age when so many other disorders had been traced to biological malfunctions, it was not difficult for physicians to conclude that an illness without consistent markers, such as neurasthenia or CFS, was an expression of a psychiatric condition. Once the leading physicians began to devalue neurasthenia as a psychiatric disorder, these patients may have been less likely to seek out medical services.

During this period, unexplained fatiguing illnesses also occurred in clustered outbreaks. Two epidemics that attracted considerable attention occurred in 1934 at the Los Angeles County Hospital and in 1955 at the Royal Free Hospital in Great Britain. Both outbreaks involved the medical staffs rather than the patients. The reported motor and sensory symptoms received diagnoses such as atypical poliomyelitis, neuromyasthenia or myalgic encephalomyelitis. Although most cases resolved within a few months, some of the affected individuals remained chronically ill with fluctuating symptoms and significant functional impairments (Briggs & Levine, 1994). Research studies were launched to better understand these outbreaks, but in general, physicians and researchers could not explain what had occurred. Because these outbreaks of acute illness affected relatively few people, they have become footnotes in medical history.

During the 1960s and 1970s, chronic brucellosis was often cited as the cause of chronic fatigue, but patients with this diagnosis were typically viewed as having psychiatric conditions, usually depression. Beginning in the mid-1980s, the term *chronic Epstein-Barr virus syndrome* was used to explain chronic fatigue as a persistent viral illness caused by the same pathogen responsible for acute mononucleosis (this link was later discredited; H. Johnson, 1995). The link between Epstein-Barr virus and CFS in the 1980s indicated a trend toward medicalization of CFS, as hundreds of articles describing this syndrome were published in medical journals over the subsequent decade.

CFS: 1980s TO THE PRESENT

In the Lake Tahoe region of Nevada, an epidemic of a mysterious disease occurred that was subsequently labeled Chronic Fatigue Syndrome by infectious disease physicians at the Centers for Disease Control (Holmes, Kaplan, Gantz, et al., 1988). A particularly poignant account of a CFS sufferer, Hillary Johnson, appeared in a 1987 issue of *Rolling Stone* magazine. As the national media discovered the illness, reports of a "new" mysterious fatiguing malady were collected from patients and physicians around the country. Hundreds of support groups were soon formed throughout the United States.

From the mid-1980s to the present, a gulf has formed between patients' perceptions of the illness and the professional response to it. In general, patients have viewed this illness as a serious and disabling consequence of some infectious agent, whereas medical personnel have explained the condition as a reversible psychiatric disorder or simply a non-illness.

Ironically, CFS in the 1990s brings us back full-circle to the medical disagreements early in this century over the nature of neurasthenia. The controversy over "mind versus body" remains at the heart of the debate. Skeptical and stigmatizing attitudes toward CFS patients have characterized the majority view in the current debate. Now that we have looked into the past, we turn to the damaging cultural milieu that affects many CFS patients in the 1990s.

CFS Onset and Stigmatization

The psychological shock of CFS onset combined with the experience of social stigmatization of the illness creates an enormous burden for the patient. In order to understand these illness burdens, the central concepts of perceived energy and fatigue require explanation. Persistent fatigue may be viewed as a loss of energy. The role of perceived energy (or the lack of it) in daily functioning is profound.

> Energy is viewed as a power resource because of the vastly important role it plays biologically, psychologically, cognitively,

and socially. Energy provides power in the following ways: It is a resource for mobility, a factor in promoting well-being and a feeling of physical reserve, a means of providing confidence in task accomplishment, and a means of responding to unexpected stress. An energy deficit contributes to powerlessness. When the capacity to do work is lacking, powerlessness exists. (Miller, 1992, p. 195)

The onset of severe fatigue and the resulting feelings of powerlessness are the first alarms experienced in CFS. Patients will initially visit a physician to get an explanation and an effective treatment for their sudden symptoms and limitations. In the most dramatic cases, a healthy, high-functioning individual may become severely disabled and perhaps bedridden from one day to the next without apparent cause. The abrupt onset of the illness will trigger fear, bewilderment, and frustration. In a descriptive study of 110 persons with CFS who completed quality of life questionnaires and interviews (Anderson & Ferrans, 1997), it was found that the illness engendered "profound and multiple losses in jobs, relationships, financial security, future plans, daily routine, hobbies, stamina and spontaneity" (p. 362). One patient in this study described the life changes associated with CFS as follows: "It's changed absolutely everything I do; what I eat, where I live. It's stopped my life. My whole perception of life, which took 30 years to put together, is totally gone" (Anderson & Ferrans, 1997, p. 363).

Because the physician usually finds no medical explanation for the fatigue symptoms (based on the negative results of the physical examination and routine laboratory tests), the patient will most likely be reassured that they are "OK" or that nothing is wrong with them. The physician, feeling obliged to explain the patient's depression-like symptoms, may also state, "You are just depressed" and suggest a psychiatric consultation. The person with CFS may perceive a condescending tone from the physician who appears to be categorizing the patient as "nuts" and thereby dismissing his or her complaints.

In a survey of a CFS self-help organization, 57% of the respondents reported being treated badly or very badly by physicians (David, Wessely, & Pelosi, 1991). Furthermore, a recent questionnaire study of 609 patients with a self-identified diagnosis of CFS (Twemlow, Bradshaw, Coyne, & Lerma, 1997) found that 66% of the respondents were reportedly made worse by their doctor's care, as compared with 22% of general medical patients (Twemlow, Bradshaw, Coyne, & Lerma, 1995). Because of widespread professional and public disbelief of their illness, individuals with CFS are highly sensitive to skeptical attitudes that might delegitimize their suffering (Gurwitt et al., 1992; McKenzie, Dechene, Friedberg, & Fontanetta, 1995; N. Ware, 1993).

Physician skeptics, such as Shorter (1995), view CFS as a cultural invention perpetuated by hypochondriacal patients, misguided physicians, and the gullible media.

> Virtually all [CFS patients are] medically well individuals in the grips of the delusion that they [are ill]. Supposed new diseases such as CFS flourish in the subcultures of hypochondriasis that form within patient support groups. The caregivers themselves contribute to their patients' somatic fixations, plunging youthful and productive people into careers of disability. In every large community there will be found at least one physician willing to play up to his patients' psychological need for organicity. The mainline press has picked up [and often endorsed] these goofy illness attributions. (Shorter, 1995, pp. 116–118)

Perceptions of stigmatization have also been associated with depression in fibromyalgia (Greenberg, Siegel, Hatcher, Dowling, & Bateman-Cass, 1996), a poorly understood condition similar to CFS. Similarly, other fatiguing illnesses, including Lyme disease and multiple sclerosis (MS), have been viewed with extreme skepticism by physicians before etiologic factors were discovered (H. Johnson, 1995; Ray, 1991). As stated by Bearn and Wessely (1994):

> There remains a tendency to denigrate these [CFS] subjects unlucky enough to have negative results . . . or whose illnesses are not accompanied by evidence of organicity, as being "psychogenic" and hence of little concern. The dismissal and lack of respect shown to patients whose distress does not conform to simple medical explanation can have consequences as malign as any of the alterations in neuroendocrine function. (p. 87)

For those patients who suffer the psychological and physical effects of stigmatization, sensitive and informed clinical intervention (see chap. 9 in this book) can help to ameliorate this type of distress. We now turn to the definition of CFS, a construct that is currently based on self-report symptom criteria.

Defining CFS

The original case definition of CFS, published in Holmes, Kaplan, Gantz, et al. (1988), described CFS as the "new onset of persistent or relapsing, debilitating fatigue . . . severe enough to reduce or impair average daily activity below 50% of the patient's premorbid activity level for a period of at least six months" (p. 388). Other conditions that might produce similar symptoms were excluded. In addition, a person had to have 8 or more of the 11 minor symptoms (e.g., sore throat,

EXHIBIT 1.1

Current U.S. Case Definition of Chronic Fatigue Syndrome

1.) Medically unexplained chronic fatigue, experienced for at least six months, which is of new or definite onset, that is not substantially alleviated by rest, that is not the result of ongoing exertion, and that results in substantial reduction in occupational, educational, social, and personal activities. Anxiety disorders, somatoform disorders, and nonpsychotic or nonmelancholic depression are not exclusionary.

The following conditions, if present, exclude a diagnosis of CFS: Past or current major depression with melancholic or psychotic features, delusional disorders, bipolar disorders, schizophrenia, anorexia nervosa, bulimia, or alcohol or substance abuse within 2 years before the onset of CFS or anytime afterward.

2.) Concurrent occurrence of 4 or more of the following symptoms, which must be persistent or recurrent during six or more months of the illness and do not predate the fatigue:
   1. Self-reported persistent or recurrent impairment in short-term memory or concentration severe enough to cause substantial reductions in previous levels of occupational, educational, social, or personal activities.
   2. Sore throat.
   3. Tender cervical or axillary lymph nodes.
   4. Muscle pain.
   5. Multiple joint pain without joint swelling or redness.
   6. Headaches of a new type, pattern, or severity.
   7. Unrefreshing sleep.
   8. Postexertional malaise lasting more than 24 hours.

From "The Chronic Fatigue Syndrome: A Comprehensive Approach to Its Definition and Study," by K. Fukuda, S. E. Straus, I. Hickie, M. C. Sharpe, J. G. Dobbins, and A. Komaroff, 1994, *Annals of Internal Medicine, 121*, pp. 953–959. Copyright 1994 by the American College of Physicians. Adapted with permission.

painful lymph nodes, unexplained generalized muscle weakness). A key problem with these original CFS criteria was the requirement of 8 or more minor symptoms, which included many unexplained somatic complaints. High numbers of unexplained somatic complaints are also common among individuals with psychiatric problems (Straus, 1992). Thus, the diagnostic criteria for CFS may have inadvertently selected subgroups of patients with high levels of psychiatric diagnoses.

In the United States, there was considerable dissatisfaction with the original Holmes, Kaplan, Gantz, et al. (1988) case definition because of the symptom overlap with psychiatric disorders, as noted above, and the inconsistent application of the definition by researchers. In 1994, a new CFS definition was published (Fukuda et al., 1994). Exhibit 1.1 presents the criteria for this new case definition. As in the old case definition, an individual must experience at least 6 months of chronic fatigue to fit the diagnosis. However, this new case definition requires only four minor symptoms (Fukuda et al., 1994), whereas the previous definition required eight minor symptoms (Holmes, Kaplan, Gantz, et al., 1988).

Although these new criteria may not bias a CFS diagnosis with as many psychiatric symptoms as the original definition, the new definition of CFS may still fail to exclude people who have purely psychosocial, stress, or psychiatric reasons for their fatigue (K. Fukuda, personal communication, August 30, 1995). In broadening the CFS definition, it is important to ensure that those patients with primary psychiatric disorders are not included within the CFS rubric (Jason, Richman, et al., 1997). The misidentification of primary psychiatric conditions as CFS could have detrimental consequences for the interpretation of both epidemiological and treatment efficacy studies.

Several additional problems should be noted with the current Fukuda et al. (1994) CFS definition:

1. The Fukuda definition does not define new or definite onset. It is important to clarify exactly what a new or definite onset means. If a person were slowly getting sick over an 8-year period, from age 27 to 35, would this case be included as a new onset? Individuals who do not have this undefined new or definite onset of CFS are excluded. Rather than exclude those who do not have a new or definite onset, it might have been better to subclassify these cases for further research.

2. The definition appears to inaccurately generalize relationships between fatigue and activity to all CFS patients, as follows: (a) The case criteria stipulate that the fatigue is not substantially alleviated by rest. However, some patients report that if they engage in only a few activities with rest intervals, minimal fatigue is experienced. It is only after engaging in high-exertion activities that overwhelming fatigue is experienced. (b) The case definition further stipulates that the fatigue is not the result of ongoing exertion. Yet some patients report that fatigue is experienced only after minimal exertion. Thus, the definition needs to clarify the relationships between rest, activity, and fatigue.

3. Finally, it is unclear what "predating the fatigue" means in the definition. The current definition requires that the four or more minor symptoms required for a diagnosis of CFS must not predate the fatigue. Thus, the definition suggests that if a patient had only four minor symptoms, and one of the symptoms (sore throat) began 5 months before the debilitating fatigue, then this individual would be excluded from a CFS diagnosis. This lack of precision in the definitional criteria will lead to problems in interrater reliability (Jason, Richman, et al., 1997).

In sum, the criteria used in the case definition have not been clearly operationalized. Field tests need to be conducted to determine the reliability and validity of these nosologies. In the determination of psychiatric diagnosis, considerable improvements were made to the subsequent editions of the *Diagnostic and Statistical Manual* (*DSM*) when committees were appointed to make recommendations concerning different features of the overall diagnostic system. These recommendations were implemented in nationwide field trials to establish diagnostic reliability. This approach might be used to bring greater precision to the current case definition of CFS (Fukuda et al., 1994), which is based on a single consensus panel of CFS researchers.[1]

The Scope of the Problem

DEMOGRAPHIC CHARACTERISTICS OF PEOPLE WITH CFS

Most studies of CFS have found few minority group members (Gunn, Connell, & Randall, 1993) and few men with CFS (Gunn et al., 1993; Manu, Lane, & Matthews, 1992b), although several atypical reports have indicated higher rates of afflicted minorities (Alisky, Iczkowski, & Foti, 1991; D. Buchwald et al., 1995; Steele et al., in press) and men (Lloyd et al., 1990). The Lloyd et al. study reported that 56% of their patients were female, whereas Lawrie and Pelosi (1995) and D. Buchwald et al. (1995) found a roughly equal number of men and women. Because women do seek health care services more often than men, it is unclear whether women have higher rates of CFS or are just more visible within the health care system (Richman, Flaherty, & Rospenda, 1994).

In addition, most studies have found CFS clinical samples to be well educated (Manu, Lane, & Matthews, 1992b) or high achievers (Shafran, 1991), although Lloyd et al. (1990) reported that 53% of their sample had occupations such as unskilled laborers and truck drivers, whereas only 14% were professionals. As Shafran (1991) has observed, high achievers who are assertive may be less likely to accept medical assurance that nothing is wrong just because the laboratory tests are normal.

Some of the discrepancies in these gender and minority rates might be attributable to the different ways that patients have been recruited for research studies. The next section will examine this issue.

---

[1] Two other case definitions, one from Great Britain (Sharpe et al., 1991) and the other from Australia (Lloyd, Hickie, Boughton, Spencer, & Wakefield, 1990) have also been proposed (see Appendix A). None of the current definitions have been empirically derived or prospectively contrasted with one another (Jason, Wagner, et al., 1995). We will use the Fukuda et al. (1994) case definition, as it is the most widely used by CFS researchers.

PREVALENCE OF CFS

Is CFS a rare illness? Or perhaps, is it a much more common condition that is misdiagnosed and therefore underreported? To begin to answer these questions, we will look critically at the early and more recent epidemiological studies. Fatigue is common in the general population, reported by 19–28% of the population (Kroenke, Wood, Mangelsdorff, Meier, & Powell, 1988). However, severe fatigue is less common, and CFS is even rarer, because most patients do not meet the key markers (i.e., 6 or more months of fatigue, no exclusionary disorders). It is possible that 5% of a community sample would have significant fatigue for 6 months (Jason, Taylor, et al., 1995; Pawlikowska et al., 1994; Price, North, Wessely, & Fraser, 1992). Yet only a small proportion of this 5% is likely to have CFS (Jason, Fitzgibbon, Taylor, Taylor, et al., 1993).

In 1994, the Centers for Disease Control (CDC) published a brochure entitled "The Facts about CFS," which estimated the prevalence of CFS to be from 4 to 10 cases per 100,000 (indicating that fewer than 19,000 adults in the United States had CFS). These rates, suggesting that CFS is a rare disorder, contrast with the unusually high number of telephone calls (up to 3,000 a month) that the CDC had been receiving from people requesting information about CFS (McCluskey, 1993). If CFS epidemiological studies had in fact substantially underestimated the number of people afflicted with this illness, the public health response to this disorder would have been inadequate.

The first widely publicized investigation of CFS epidemiology, from which the above estimates were derived, was initiated in the late 1980s by the CDC (Gunn et al., 1993). Because this study was based on physician referrals, many low-income individuals who do not have access to the health care system may have been excluded (Mechanic, 1983). Thus, it may be inappropriate to estimate prevalence solely from physicians or treatment facilities. For instance, disadvantaged minorities do manifest higher levels of chronic illness, and they are less likely to receive adequate care or be counted in epidemiological studies from treatment sources (Dutton, 1986). In addition, physicians who are skeptical of the disorder's existence will be less likely to make referrals in epidemiological studies (Richman et al., 1994).

In contrast to the preceding CDC report, a very high prevalence of CFS was found in a study of a specific occupational group. Jason and colleagues (Jason, Wagner, et al., in press) directly surveyed 3,400 nurses, of whom 6% indicated that they had experienced debilitating fatigue for 6 months or longer (Jason, Taylor, et al., 1993a, 1993b). Thirty-seven nurses met case criteria for current CFS, yielding a prevalence rate of 1,088 per 100,000 (Jason, Wagner, et al., in press), considerably higher than the CDC estimates reported above. Because nurses may be a high-risk population for CFS (e.g., nurses' work is stressful; its schedules often disrupt circadian rhythms), it may be inappropriate to generalize these data to the entire population (Grufferman, 1991).

Community Sample Studies

In 1993, Jason and colleagues (Jason, Taylor, et al., 1995) estimated rates of CFS using a completely random community sample (N = 1,031). Five percent of the sample indicated that they had experienced unexplained, severe fatigue for 6 months or more. The majority of the fatigued group indicated that they had no current medical doctor overseeing their illness. This study yielded an estimated CFS prevalence of 200 per 100,000 (Jason, Taylor, et al., 1995), a rate almost 20 times higher than the CDC figures cited earlier. In the summer of 1995, Jason and colleagues began a larger scale community-based epidemiologic investigation of CFS involving a sample of 30,000 randomly selected people. The findings will be released in the fall of 1998.

Another study that suggested similar rates to those found in the Jason, Taylor, et al. (1995) involved a random sample of 4,000 individuals on a health maintenance organization roster in the Seattle area (D. Buchwald et al., 1995). The estimated prevalence rate of CFS was 75 to 267 per 100,000. Subsequently, the CDC conducted its own community-based survey in San Francisco (Steele et al., in press). The prevalence of CFS-like disorders was estimated to be 200 per 100,000. Unfortunately, this study collected only self-report data without medical and psychiatric examinations. Based on these recent prevalence findings, epidemiologists at the CDC have recently shifted all surveillance efforts to community-based population surveys. Table 1.1 provides a summary of prevalence studies, grouped by sampling methods (i.e., physician referral, samples from health care facilities, and random community samples). The CDC has now added CFS to the list of Priority-1 New and Reemerging Infectious Diseases, indicating that CFS is now defined as a top CDC priority. (Other priority-1 diseases include *E. coli* infection and tuberculosis.)

CFS Versus Primary Depression

A final epidemiologic study, conducted in Great Britain, deserves consideration, in part because their estimated prevalence rates for CFS were much higher than any previous study. This investigation (Wessely et al., 1995) ascertained the presence of CFS in a sample of people who presented to the physician with either symptoms of

TABLE 1.1

Prevalence Studies Conducted to Date

Authors	N	Rates
Physician-identified populations		
Gunn, Connell, & Randall (1993)	408 physicians	2.0 to 7.3 per 100,000 8.6 to 15.1 per 100,000 (adjusted)
Lloyd, Hickie, Boughton, Spencer, & Wakefield (1990)	104 physicians	39.6 per 100,000
Ho-Yen & McNamara (1991)	195 physicians	130 per 100,000
Health facility populations directly surveyed		
Bates et al. (1993)	1,000 patients	300 per 100,000 (CDC criteria) 400 per 100,000 (British criteria) 1,000 per 100,000 (Australian criteria)
D. Buchwald et al. (1995)	4,000 patients	75 per 100,000 267 per 100,000 (adjusted)
Lawrie & Pelosi (1995)	1,000 patients	560 per 100,000 (British criteria)
Wessely et al. (1997)	2,366 patients	2,600 per 100,000 (Fukuda criteria)
Randomly selected populations		
Price, North, Wessely, & Fraser (1992)	13,538 respondents	7.4 per 100,000
Jason, Fitzgibbon, Taylor, Johnson, & Salina (1993)	1,031 respondents	200 per 100,000
Steele et al. (in press)	17,155 households	76 to 233 per 100,000

infections or other medical problems. A subsequent study (Wessely, Chalder, Hirsch, Wallace, & Wright, 1997) using the Fukuda et al. (1994) definition determined that 2.6% of this sample had CFS.

It is of interest that this high CFS rate, about 10 times higher than community-based estimates, is within the range of prevalence of several mood disorders. For major depressive episode, the 1-month prevalence is 2.2%, and lifetime prevalence is 5.8% (Regier et al., 1988). Seventy-four percent of the above CFS sample had a psychiatric diagnosis before the onset of their fatigue, and 59% believed that their illness might be due to psychological or psychosocial causes (Euba, Chalder, Deale, & Wessely, 1996). Yet this finding of an increased prevalence of CFS was based on the same case definition (Fukuda et al., 1994) used in recent community studies. This high prevalence estimate may indicate the inclusion of pure psychiatric cases in the category of CFS disorders.

Many symptoms of psychiatric illnesses, particularly depression, can overlap with CFS symptoms; thus, it is critically important to distinguish patients who have primary psychiatric disorders from those who have CFS. For instance, primary depression (without CFS) is one alternative explanation for persistent fatigue. Some patients with major depressive disorder (without CFS) report chronic fatigue and four minor CFS symptoms such as unrefreshing sleep, joint pain, muscle pain, and concentration difficulty. Fatigue plus these four minor symptoms also defines a case of CFS. Given this possibility of symptom overlap, some patients with a primary affective disorder might be misdiagnosed as having CFS. Our review of the data strongly suggests that the inclusion of pure psychiatric disorder, such as depression, artificially inflates prevalence estimates in epidemiologic studies of CFS. As a result, treatment studies may report deceptively high rates of remission and recovery.

Conclusions

Initial research suggested that CFS was a relatively rare disorder. However, serious methodological problems in many of the early epidemiological studies of CFS (Gunn et al., 1993; Price et al., 1992) cast doubt on these early findings. By the mid-1990s, findings from more representative epidemiologic studies indicated considerably higher CFS prevalence rates. Their findings (Bates et al., 1993; D. Buchwald et al., 1995; Jason, Taylor, et al., 1995; Lawrie & Pelosi, 1995; Steele et al., in press) suggest that there might be from 145,000 to 1,084,000 people with CFS. If the CFS definition is broadened, as reflected in a study by Wessely et al. (1995), rates of CFS might be considerably higher.

PROGNOSIS

D.S. Bell (1991) suggested that, after 2 years, about 80% of patients experience improvement that is due to a lessening of symptom severity, a loss of fear concerning the disease, or an alteration of lifestyle to accommodate functional limitations. Those with reduced symptoms may still experience exacerbations during periods of stress and minor illness. Yet relatively few patients are cured, and a significant minority of patients experience progressive worsening of symptoms. It is not uncommon for those with more severe symptoms to have suicidal thoughts or feelings (Collinge, 1993).

Prospective outcome studies of CFS indicate that improvements often occur, but recovery is rare. Wilson et al. (1994) recontacted 103 CFS patients at a 3½-year follow-up. Many remained functionally impaired, and only 6 had completely recovered. Steele, Reyes, and Dobbins (1994) followed 478 CFS patients over a mean of 23 months and found that only 36 had made a full recovery, whereas 64 reported more symptoms over time. In another longitudinal outcome study (Bombardier & Buchwald, 1995) of CFS patients contacted an average of 1.5 years after an initial evaluation, 61% reported some improvement, although an extremely small proportion of patients reported a remission of fatigue.

A recent review of CFS naturalistic outcome studies (Joyce, Hotopf, & Wessely, 1997) concluded that fewer than 10% of patients returned to premorbid levels of functioning, whereas the majority of CFS patients remained significantly impaired. The summary article further stated that the presence of psychiatric disorder and patients' belief in a physical cause for their symptoms were predictors of poor outcome. In a critique of the Joyce et al. (1997) article, Hedrick (1997) pointed out that many of the reviewed longitudinal studies on CFS prognosis used different diagnostic instruments, different definitions of improvement, and different periods of follow-up. In a discussion of the psychiatric predictors of poor outcome, Hedrick (1997) noted the following:

> Some studies found no prospective relationships; others found relationships on only one or a few of numerous factors; and different factors were found to be significant in different studies. More importantly, the strength of such relationships is often so low as to be of little significance in either understanding the etiology of CFS or guiding its treatment. (p. 725)

In contrast to the above outcome studies, Camacho and Jason (1997) found few differences between 15 recovered and 15 nonrecovered people with CFS on a wide range of psychosocial factors. The only significant differences between the recovered and nonrecovered groups were on fatigue and symptom measures, which suggests that organic variables have an etiologic role in the illness.

Despite an emerging research literature suggesting that CFS has both biological and psychiatric aspects, many physicians, media professionals, and lay people continue to believe that CFS is a purely psychiatric phenomenon or a form of malingering to gain attention and sympathy. It is our hope that this book will promote an understanding of CFS as a complex and persistent illness. As this understanding develops, researchers and clinicians will construct better working models to assess and treat the underserved population of CFS sufferers.

Overview of the Book

This book provides a review and synthesis of psychological, behavioral, and biological variables associated with CFS. These complementary themes of review and synthesis are reflected in each of the three parts of this volume: overview, assessment, and treatment.

In chapter 2, we focus on predisposing factors and explore why certain individuals may be more likely to develop the illness than others. Assessing and evaluating predisposing factors will allow the clinician and the researcher to better understand the heterogeneous etiology of the syndrome, to better differentiate between correlational and causal factors, and to better treat individuals who present highly diverse medical and psychiatric histories.

We present in chapter 3 four explanatory models of CFS and then review relevant data from psychoneuroimmunology in relation to CFS. These models range in their conceptualizations of the illness from a purely cultural phenomenon to a more biologically based view. In chapter 4, we review CFS symptom assessment and propose a new, more refined system of evaluation to assess and rate symptom severity in diagnostic procedures.

We critically evaluate fatigue rating scales in chapter 5, including fatigue intensity scales, fatigue/function measures, and fatigue/affect assessments. The chapter concludes with recommendations for clinicians and researchers concerning the use of fatigue scales. In chapter 6, we examine psychometric instruments in CFS assessment, including measures of depression, functional status, psychiatric status (or well-being), coping, social support, locus-of-control, subjective pain, somatic perception, and illness behavior and attribution. In addition, we describe a suggested comprehensive assessment protocol.

Chapter 7 addresses diagnostic issues. In this chapter, we offer guidelines for the differential diagnosis of CFS in relation to depression, somatization disorder, generalized anxiety disorder, stress symptoms, and Axis II disorders. Non-CFS chronic fatigue is distinguished from CFS, as are a variety of overlap syndromes, including postinfectious Lyme disease, fibromyalgia, multiple chemical sensitivities, and irritable bowel syndrome.

Medical and alternative therapies are the focus of chapter 8, whereas in chapter 9, we review cognitive–behavioral therapy outcome studies and presents an overall coping skills treatment approach for the CFS patient. In chapter 10, we provide a transcript of a psychological interview with a CFS patient, along with interspersed clinical observations about assessment, diagnosis, and treatment. Next, a formalized coping skills intervention for CFS groups is presented with step-by-step instructions in chapter 11. The final chapter (12) documents the service needs of CFS patients and the community-based interventions that might prove effective with this population.

Because this volume is written for the mental health professional, we focus on psychological, psychosocial, and behavioral aspects of CFS, with an emphasis on assessment and treatment. An important secondary focus of this book, medical and biological aspects of the illness—including predisposing biological factors (chap. 2), biological models (chap. 3), medical therapies (chap. 8), and medical assessment (Appendix B), are presented using language that can be understood by both the medical and nonmedical professional. Thus, the reader is exposed to the full range of research and clinical data on CFS, combined with pertinent patient narratives and case histories to help the reader understand this complex illness.

Predisposing Factors

2

Why do certain individuals seem to be more prone to develop this illness than others? Psychosocial factors may be one important influence in the development of CFS. This chapter examines predisposing factors in order to better understand the heterogeneous etiology of this syndrome and to better differentiate between correlational and causal factors. The ultimate goal of this type of analysis is to develop treatments for individuals who present highly diverse medical and psychiatric histories. We will first consider the influences of stress and coping, personality, and biological factors in the etiology of CFS, and then review studies that compare somatization disorder, depression, and other medical conditions with CFS.

Stress and Coping

Several researchers have found that stress and coping styles are related to illness and immune function (Cohen & Williamson, 1991). For instance, Meyer and Haggarty (1962) found that infectious diseases caused by common bacteria such as streptococcus have been related to both acute and chronic stress. Furthermore, individuals with heightened catecholamine and cardiovascular reactions to stress are more likely to show suppression in their immune functions in response to a 20-minute laboratory stressor

(Manuck, Cohen, Rabin, Muldoon, & Bachen, 1991). Viral illness may also be related to stress and coping factors. For example, in a study of mononucleosis among cadets (Kasl, Evans, & Niederman, 1979), infected (vs. noninfected) cadets were found to be very committed to military careers and had fathers who were described as overachievers. Yet these cadets performed poorly in academic subjects. These cadets were therefore likely experiencing high stress.

These illustrative studies suggest that stress and coping styles might increase susceptibility to infectious diseases; at the present time, however, there is no definitive evidence linking psychological states to specific diseases of the immune system (Bower, 1991).

Personality Factors

Some investigators have studied the relationships between personality factors and fatigue states or prolonged recovery from illness (Abbey, 1993). In an early study of personality and illness, Imboden, Canter, and Cluff (1961) prospectively evaluated military personnel before an Asian influenza epidemic. Of the 26 people who became ill, the 12 who had not recovered at a 3- to 6-week follow-up had higher premorbid levels of emotional disturbance and depressive vulnerability.

Studies of personality factors in chronic fatigue have also been reported. Montgomery (1983) found that individuals with complaints of chronic fatigue in the absence of infection had higher levels of introversion and neuroticism. In a more recent study comparing CFS patients with chronic pain patients and healthy controls (Blakely et al.,1991), no unique psychological characteristics were identified as antecedents or consequences of CFS, although the authors concluded that high levels of emotionality and neuroticism may act as predisposing factors. Finally, in a correlational study (Cope, David, Pelosi, & Mann, 1994) of fatigue and psychosocial variables, a less definite diagnosis by a general practitioner and the tendency of the patient to attribute symptoms to physical disorders rather than to psychological factors were significant predictors of chronic fatigue.

Biological Factors

Biological antecedents may also play a role in CFS. Lanham and Lanham (1994) found more autoimmune diseases in families of CFS patients than in healthy controls. Autoimmune diseases are partly the result of genetic predisposition, so it is possible that people with CFS have inherited a genetic predisposition to immunologic diseases and perhaps to CFS. In another family study, Abbot et al. (1996) found CD38 immune activation markers raised in most CFS patients, as well as in their household contacts. Because this particular immune marker is associated with viral infection, it may be that the infective agent is resisted by the healthy family member, whereas the CFS patient succumbs to the illness.

Several studies have also reported cardiovascular abnormalities in patients with CFS. An investigation by Cordero et al. (1996) found no significant differences between patients with CFS and healthy controls on mean heart rate, tidal volume, minute volume, respiratory rate, oxygen consumption, or total spectrum power. However, after periods of walking, a subtle abnormality was detected in vagal activity (a noninvasive index of parasympathetic influence) to the heart in patients with CFS; this could, in part, account for postexertional symptom exacerbation.

Somatization Disorder and Attribution

Somatization has been proposed as a partial explanation for CFS symptoms. Katon and Walker (1993) found that the prevalence of somatization disorder in CFS patients averages 10–15%, at least three times higher than in other medical populations. Somatization, defined as one or more medically unexplained symptoms, is presumably related to underlying emotional or social difficulties. Somatizing patients avoid the blame that would be associated with a psychological attribution by focusing on bodily symptoms (Goldberg & Bridges, 1988). For instance, Wessely and Powell (1989) found that 86% of patients with postviral fatigue attributed their illness to physical factors, whereas only 14% of depressive patients attributed their illness to such factors.

Poor outcomes for CFS patients in a longitudinal outcome study (Wilson et al., 1994) and in cognitive–behavioral therapy treatment programs (Butler, Chalder, Ron, & Wessely, 1991; Sharpe et al., 1996) have also been associated with patient attribution of physical causes for CFS. These studies suggest that individuals with CFS attribute their illness to external causes and that such attributions might help them avoid self-blame. However, most of this research used the Holmes, Kaplan, Gantz, et al. (1988) definition of CFS, which requires eight or more minor symptoms. Thus, individuals might have been selected who had a higher likelihood of having somatization and other psychiatric disorders (Katon & Russo, 1992). In addition, if CFS symptoms are biologically based, then these symptoms reflect a true medical illness rather than somatization.

Other investigations of CFS symptomatology have not supported a somatization model. A recent study (Wood, Bentall, Gopfert, Dewey, & Edwards, 1994) that exposed chronic fatigue patients to a stressful task found no evidence for the hypothesis that CFS participants respond to stress with physical rather than psychological symptoms. In addition, Ray, Weir, Cullen, and Phillips (1992) found no significant relation between indices of perceived CFS illness severity (e.g, frequency of symptoms, course of illness, disability, severity of illness) and emotional distress. The absence of a relationship between these two variables may be one reason why people with CFS attribute their illness to physical rather than psychological causes.

Finally, if people with CFS present physical complaints in order to mask their psychological problems, then an inverse relationship should exist between the number of depression and anxiety symptoms, and the number of reported somatic symptoms (Katon & Walker, 1993). However, this relationship has not been found; rather, people who become distressed report more somatic, depression, and anxiety symptoms concurrently (Katon & Russo, 1992; Katon & Walker, 1993).

CFS Versus Depression

Fatigue is one of the most common presenting symptoms of depression (Thase, 1991). Because fatigue is present in all cases of CFS, some have suggested that depression might be the cause of CFS. Although an early comparative study of CFS and primary depression (Wessely & Powell, 1989) showed considerable symptomatic overlap between the two disorders, a number of subsequent studies have suggested that CFS is distinct from depression in both biological and psychiatric domains.

Several studies of brain pathology have revealed differences between CFS and depression. CFS patients show more alpha electroencephalographic (EEG) activity during non–rapid eye movement (NREM) sleep, a condition that is not seen in dysthymic or major depressive disorders (Whelton, Salit, & Moldofsky, 1992). Other EEG abnormalities have been found in CFS that are not reflections of major depression. In comparison with patients with depression, individuals with CFS show more frequent spike waves, sharp waves, high amplitude alpha waves, and more frequent bursts of theta waves (Donati, Fagioli, Komaroff, & Duffy, 1994). In a recent investigation, Samii et al. (1996) reported that the facilitation of motor-evoked potentials in patients with CFS was reduced in a first postexercise period, whereas this was not the case with depressed patients. This means that postexercise cortical excitability is significantly reduced in patients with CFS. Contrary to the above findings, Cope, Pernet, Kendall, and David (1995) did not find significant differences in brain pathology (white matter lesions) based on magnetic resonance imaging between a sample of fatigued patients, most of whom met the criteria for CFS, and a psychiatric depressed sample.

Neurological and immunological findings also indicate differences between CFS and depression. Bakheit, Behan, Dinan, Gray, and O'Keane (1992) found upregulation of hypothalamic 5-hydroxytryptamine receptors in patients with postviral fatigue syndrome but not in those with primary depression. These receptors have been linked to several hypothalamic functions, including sleep, appetite, mood, memory, and temperature regulation. Furthermore, Cleare et al. (1995) found that depression was associated with hypercotisolaemia and reduced central 5-HT neurotransmission, whereas CFS was associated with hypocotisolaemia and reduced central 5-HT neurotransmission. Also, baseline cortisol levels (and prolactin responses) were highest in the depressed group, lowest in the CFS group, and intermediate between the two in the healthy control group. These findings point to biological distinctions between these disorders.

Another biological study (Lutgendorf, Klimas, et al., 1995) pointed to a relationship between immunological function and cognitive deficits in CFS. When depression was statistically controlled in CFS, those patients with greater cognitive difficulties showed more abnormalities in their immune system (Lutgendorf, Klimas, et al., 1995). This finding suggests that the presence of cognitive difficulties in CFS patients cannot be explained solely by mood disturbances.

The psychiatric status of CFS and of depressed patients also appears to be different. Pepper, Krupp, Friedberg, Doscher, and Coyle (1993) reported clear differences between CFS patients and patients with major depression; that is, CFS patients had a lower incidence of schizoid, avoidant, passive–aggressive, and self-defeating personality disorders and a lower level of depressive symptoms. In another comparative study of CFS and depression (Hickie, Lloyd, Wakefield, & Parker, 1990), 90% of primary depression patients showed premorbid psychiatric diagnoses, whereas only 24.5% of the CFS group had premorbid psychiatric disorders. These rates for CFS patients are similar to that of the general population, although Abbey and

Garfinkel (1991a) have raised several questions about potentially confounding factors in this study. Finally, Shanks and Ho-Yen (1995) evaluated CFS at a secondary referral center, where patients tend to receive treatment for more recent illness. They found the prevalence of current psychiatric disorders to be 45%, which is similar to that found with medical patients, while premorbid prevalence rates were 17%, a figure comparable to epidemiologic studies of community samples.

CFS and Psychiatric Comorbidity

Other researchers have reported much higher psychiatric rates in CFS samples. For example, Taerk, Toner, Salit, Garfinkel, and Ozersky (1987) found that 50% of patients with neuromyasthenia (CFS) had a history of at least one major depressive episode before illness onset. In a later study (Kruesi, Dale, & Straus, 1989), 75% of CFS patients had a lifetime prevalence of psychiatric problems, and 26 of the 28 patients acquired chronic fatigue after the onset of psychiatric disorders. A limitation in this study is that all participants had unusual Epstein-Barr virus (EBV) serology profiles. Allen and Tilkian (1986) have suggested that the intensity of depressive symptoms is positively correlated with immune response to EBV infection. In addition, both the Taerk et al. (1987) and Kruesi et al. (1989) studies selected patients from tertiary care clinics. Such patients often have increased health care utilization and higher rates of somaticized depression.

Several subsequent studies have also reported high rates of psychiatric comorbidity. Wessely and Powell (1989) evaluated patients with postviral fatigue syndrome, finding that 72% evidenced lifetime psychiatric disorders, whereas 47% were diagnosed with major depression. Similarly, Gold et al. (1990) reported that 42% of tertiary care patients with CFS met criteria for current major depressive episode, whereas 50% had experienced major depression before the onset of chronic fatigue. Two other studies (Katon, Buchwald, Simon, Russo, & Mease, 1991; Lane, Manu, & Matthews, 1991) found extremely high rates of lifetime depression (75–77%), and 43% of the sample in the latter report had experienced episodes of depression at least 1 year before the onset of CFS.

Reporting somewhat lower psychiatric rates, the CDC prevalence study found that 58% of their sample had psychological problems prior to, during, or after the onset of fatigue (Gunn et al., 1993). Also, a recent study by MacDonald, Osterholm, LeDell, White, and Schenk,

(1996) reported no significant premorbid history of depression in a sample of healthy controls or in a group diagnosed with CFS, although those with CFS were more likely to have a diagnosis of depression subsequent to the onset of CFS.

The high prevalence of psychodiagnoses in the aforementioned studies may be explained in part by the case selection criteria. Many of the studies reviewed used a definition of CFS that required eight or more minor symptoms. This high symptom frequency threshold might have inadvertently selected individuals with a greater likelihood of psychiatric disorders such as depression and somatization (Katon & Russo, 1992). In addition, people ill with CFS often experience generalized emotional distress that may be evidenced as a greater number of psychiatric complaints. Such symptoms may better be considered a single dimension of reactive distress rather than a self-contained clinical diagnosis (Ray, 1991).

Another methodological problem is the use of idiosyncratic selection criteria for CFS that may yield inaccurate estimates of psychiatric morbidity. Manu and associates (Manu, Lane, & Matthews, 1988; Manu, Matthews, & Lane, 1988; Manu et al., 1989) used an exercise stress test, an activity that few individuals currently meeting a formal criteria definition of CFS could perform. In addition, these researchers selected patients with only mild occupational impairments (only two patients in the Manu study missed work because of illness in the year preceding the evaluation). Thus, it is unlikely that the results from such research can be generalized to the majority of the CFS population.

In contrast to the preceding data, three comparative studies of CFS, MS, and depression (see Table 2.1; S. K. Johnson, DeLuca, & Natelson, 1996b; Natelson et al., 1995; Pepper et al., 1993) found that participants with CFS more closely resembled MS patients than they did clinical depression patients on measures of somatic and psychiatric symptoms, including fatigue severity. MS may be an ideal medical comparison group for CFS because generalized, disabling fatigue is a prominent symptom (Pepper et al., 1993). In addition, Stone et al. (1994) recently found, using in vivo assessments, that CFS patients did not differ from nonpatients in overall levels of positive and negative affectivity. This finding argues against an explanation of CFS as a form of depression.

Based on prior psychodiagnostic studies, David et al. (1991) concluded that depression occurs in about 50% of CFS cases and that anxiety and somatization disorders (including somatization, minor depression, phobia, anxiety disorders, and conversion disorders) occur in about 25% of cases. It is still unclear whether these high psychiatric rates are a cause, an effect, or a covariate of CFS. It is important to remember, as Krupp, Mendelson, and Friedman (1991) noted, that 25–35% of patients have no psychiatric condition. The size of this

TABLE 2.1

Comparative Studies

Authors	Samples	Findings
Wessely & Powell (1989)	CFS, neuromuscular fatiguing illness, major depression	CFS & affective groups—more physical and mental fatigue; more psychiatric diagnoses. Neuromuscular group—less mental fatigue, fewer psychiatric diagnoses.
Krupp, Mendelson, & Friedman (1991) Pepper et al. (1993)	CFS, MS, systemic lupus erythematosus (SLE), Lyme disease, primary depression and controls	CFS and MS similar in fatigue and psychopathology, but depression more frequent in CFS group following onset of illness. MS group—greater cognitive impairment. CFS group—higher fatigue and fewer psychiatric diagnoses than depression group.
DeLuca, Johnson, Beldowicz, & Natelson (1995) S. K. Johnson, DeLuca, & Natelson (1996c) Natelson et al. (1995)	CFS, depression, MS, controls	Nondepressed CFS subgroup— deficit in complex attention. Depressed group—more severe psychopathology.
Packer, Sauriol, & Brouwer (1994)	CFS, MS, controls	CFS & MS groups—higher levels of fatigue, reduced activity levels, and lower perceived health status.
Komaroff et al. (1996)	CF, MS, depression, controls	Severe debilitating fatigue in 100% (CF), 80% (MS), & 28% (depression). CF group differs from other two groups on the following symptoms: mylagias, postexertional malaise, headaches, and infectious type symptoms.

Note: CF = chronic fatigue; CFS = chronic fatigue syndrome; MS = multiple sclerosis.

subgroup suggests that CFS cannot be completely attributable to psychological factors.

Differentiating CFS samples by psychiatric comorbidity is a crucial task for both researchers and clinicians. One emerging area of investigation that may empirically distinguish CFS patients with and without psychiatric disturbance is neuropsychological testing. For example, in CFS patients who are depressed, performance deficits have been found on a naturalistic task about which they complain (reading), whereas these deficits have not been found on the same type of task for nondepressed patients with CFS (Wearden & Appleby, 1997). When a more traditional laboratory test of memory (a paired associate learning test) was used, no differences were found between CFS and healthy control samples. Thus, the documentation of the ubiquitous memory and concentration complaints reported by CFS samples may require differentiation by psychiatric status and the assessment of deficits using more naturalistic methods.

CFS Versus Other Medical Disorders

Studies that have compared CFS with other medical disorders are reviewed in Table 2.1. In general, the findings indicate that (a) CFS and multiple sclerosis groups evidence higher levels of fatigue and lower levels of activity than do healthy controls (Komaroff et al., 1996; Krupp et al., 1991; Packer, Sauriol, & Brouwer, 1994); (b) CFS groups have more difficulties in processing information (DeLuca, Johnson, Beldowicz, & Natelson, 1995); and (c) MS groups have overall higher levels of cognitive dysfunction (Krupp, Sliwinski, Masur, Friedberg, & Coyle, 1994).

Conclusion

Many individuals with CFS have had psychiatric problems before or after CFS onset, although some individuals with CFS have not experienced psychiatric problems. Those patients who were depressed prior to CFS onset may have had vulnerable coping strategies and support systems. Coping deficits and persistent depressive states might have negatively influenced their immune systems and, as a consequence, placed them at higher risk of developing CFS. Those without pre-existing psychiatric disorders who develop CFS might experience illness-related depression and other psychiatric disorders associated with the loss of work and social roles. Furthermore, negative coping strategies and reactive mood disorders might hamper efforts toward recovery. Individuals with CFS who do not experience psychiatric disorders after onset of CFS may still endure profound negative effects on their social networks and coping capacities, which might in turn influence the recovery process. Stress, social support, coping styles, and psychiatric comorbidity may be important mediators for understanding disease onset and maintenance.

Explanatory Models of Chronic Fatigue Syndrome

3

n order to understand an illness as complex and heterogeneous as CFS, one must juggle and blend theoretical information from a variety of disciplines. Specifically, immunological, neurological, and psychological factors may interact in ways that call for a comprehensive theoretical approach. In addition, the diagnostic confusion between CFS and other disorders, and the possibility that more than one disorder might actually exist under the CFS rubric, make it all the more important to take a careful and discriminating approach toward new and existing research.

The models of CFS presented below are considerably varied in their emphasis, ranging from a purely biological conceptualization of the illness at one extreme to a sociocultural hypothesis at the other. Although the mind–body dichotomy has exerted a strong influence over how CFS is viewed—that is, as either a psychiatric or medical illness (N. C. Ware, 1993)—the literature on CFS strongly suggests that the illness involves both biological and psychiatric aspects. Given the diversity of CFS, the influence of biological and psychiatric factors may differ substantially within the CFS population. Thus, these models may accurately characterize the illness for one subgroup of patients but not another. Yet each may offer insights into the pathogenesis of this debilitating illness.

Four explanatory models of CFS will be described: (a) an immune activation model that views CFS symptoms as caused by chronic overactivation of the immune system;

(b) a symptom avoidance model that conceptualizes the illness as triggered by a transitory acute infection, but maintained by psychological factors; (c) an illness reactivity model that interprets psychological disorders as secondary reactions to a biological illness; and (d) a conversion model that views psychological factors as the primary cause of the syndrome. Finally, research findings in psychoneuroimmunology, which may form the basis of a future biopsychosocial model of the illness, are presented and integrated with published CFS data.

Immune Activation Model

Straus, Dale, Wright, and Metcalfe (1988) have proposed that the underlying disorder causing CFS, viral infections, psychiatric disorders, and allergies is a chronic overactivation of the immune system that produces persistent flu-like symptoms. Such flu-like symptoms (e.g., sore throat, fatigue, headache) are normally associated with transitory acute illnesses and then disappear once the pathogenic agent has been subdued by immune defenses. According to the model, however, the immune response in CFS remains elevated despite the absence of an identified disease-producing agent.

In a review of the literature, Patarca, Fletcher, and Klimas (1993) summarized evidence for chronic immune activation in CFS, which includes elevations of activated T lymphocytes, and poor cellular function as represented by natural killer (NK) cell cytotoxicity and frequent immunoglobulin deficiencies (most often IgG1 and IgG3).[1] Typical of the research supporting immunological problems is that of Landay, Jessop, Lennette, and Levy (1991), who found in CFS patients that the CD8 CD11b suppressor cell population was reduced, while the activation markers (CD38 and HLA-DR) were elevated. These findings suggest that decreased suppressor cells lead to a hyperimmune response. Such immune activation might trigger increases in cytokines that are associated with fatigue and other symptoms of viral infections.

Deficits in cortisol, a stress-related neuro-hormone, have also been linked to lethargy and fatigue, and this deficit might contribute to an overactive immune system. A well-known study by Demitrack, Dale, Straus, Lane, and Listwak, (1991) found low levels of cortisol in CFS patients, which might be due to a deficit of corticotropin-releasing

---

[1]Immunoglobulins are antibodies that respond to foreign invaders. There are five types of these antibodies. One type is called IgG antibodies, which appear later in the immune response. Another type, IgM antibodies, appear early in the immune response.

hormone. Similar abnormalities occur in nurses who are involved in fatigue-producing night shift work (Leese et al., 1996). Wessely (1993), however, stated that it is simplistic to view CFS as solely a deficiency in corticotropin-releasing factor (CRF) and suggested, alternatively, that some abnormality in CRF metabolism may underlie both depression and CFS.

Further evidence for immune abnormalities has been reported by Straus, Fritz, Dale, Gould, and Strober (1993) who found that CFS patients have memory T-cells with increased levels of adhesion markers. These memory cells appear to shift from the blood to the tissues. Such tissue-based cells escape detection by research blood tests. The increased number of memory cells with adhesion markers in the tissues will trigger the release of molecules that regulate the immune response, which in turn can cause mild inflammation and pain. The Straus et al. (1993) findings may explain some of the complaints of CFS patients, including painful muscles and joints and tender lymph nodes. One reason for medical skepticism of CFS is that many studies examining cellular immune response abnormalities in people with CFS have not produced consistent findings (Krupp et al., 1991).

Symptom Avoidance Hypothesis

According to the symptom avoidance model (Butler et al., 1991), an acute infectious illness may cause CFS and account for symptom severity during the initial phases of the illness. As the infection subsides, however, symptom severity and disability may persist due to an established habit of activity avoidance and a phobic-like concern about preventing symptom flare-ups. This physical activation–psychological maintenance hypothesis was adapted from the chronic pain literature (Philips, 1987) and served as a framework for an initial cognitive–behavioral intervention in CFS (S. Butler et al., 1991).

An elaboration of the symptom avoidance model (Surawy, Hackmann, Hawton, & Sharpe, 1995) proposed that severe, ongoing psychosocial stressors in combination with a minor illness precipitate increasing personal efforts to meet performance targets and propel the individual into a state of chronic exhaustion, frustration, and demoralization. According to this hypothesis, the patient generates a pathological coping reaction by dwelling on the somatic symptoms of the behavioral condition and wrongly attributing them to a physical disease. As symptom preoccupation increases, disability and demoralization increase as well, resulting in a cycle of perpetuation of the illness condition.

In support of the symptom avoidance model, two controlled clinical trials of cognitive–behavioral therapy (Deale et al., 1997; Sharpe et al., 1996) and a controlled study of a physical exercise treatment (Fulcher & White, 1997), all based on graduated activity schedules (i.e., step-wise exposure), reported substantial improvements in the majority of treated CFS patients, whereas only a small minority were significantly better in the control conditions. Furthermore, a cross-sectional study of 282 CFS sufferers (Petrie, Moss-Morris, & Weinman, 1995) found that the participants who endorsed catastrophic beliefs had significantly higher levels of fatigue and disability, suggesting that maladaptive thinking may contribute to reduced functioning.

Additional evidence for the symptom avoidance model may be found in a correlational study of psychological coping and illness appraisals in CFS (Antoni et al., 1994). Symptom severity and disability were moderately associated with maladaptive coping responses, including behavioral disengagement (a form of giving up) and denial (of CFS diagnosis). These correlations suggest that poor coping may contribute to debilitation in CFS patients. The cross-sectional design of this study prohibits inferences about the direction of the relationship between maladaptive coping and illness burden.

Other data do not support the symptom avoidance model. Trigwell, Hatcher, Johnson, Stanley, and Honse (1995), in a comparative study of 90 CFS patients and 70 MS patients, found no differences in abnormal illness behavior on the Illness Behavior Questionnaire between the two groups, although both groups had significantly elevated scores on the general hypochondriasis and disease conviction subscales in relation to normative data. Rather than viewing abnormal illness behavior as "proof" of psychogenesis in CFS, these findings suggest that maladaptive illness behavior may coexist with chronic medical illness.

Finally, the Butler et al. (1991) model assumes that moderate to severe disability in CFS is due to an intensifying cycle of fear-based activity avoidance. Yet a substantial percentage of individuals with CFS report relatively high functioning. In an epidemiologic study (D. Buchwald et al., 1995), a large proportion of individuals identified with CFS or idiopathic chronic fatigue were working full-time, although they were presumably impaired in some areas such as exercise capacity and cognitive function. In the absence of comorbid phobia, depression, or other debilitating psychiatric disorder, it is not clear how the symptom avoidance model would explain the illness in these high-functioning individuals (Wessely, 1996).

Illness Reactivity Model

Alternatively, Friedberg and Krupp (1994) have proposed that primarily biological factors maintain disability and symptom severity in CFS, although such factors may trigger secondary psychological reactions in vulnerable individuals. Emotional reactions to disabling symptoms, such as depression and anxiety may be associated with additional fatigue (*DSM–IV*; American Psychiatric Association, 1994) and may increase overall fatigue severity. The perception of higher levels of burdensome fatigue, in turn, amplifies emotional distress. Figure 9.1 (see p. 139) illustrates the cycle of fatigue and emotional stress in CFS. On the other hand, pleasant emotions (e.g., elation) may interrupt the unhealthy fatigue–stress interaction, lessen the burden of symptoms and limitations, and increase the likelihood of long-term improvement (see Figure 9.2 on p. 139).

Three clinical studies (Friedberg & Krupp, 1994; Ray, Jefferies, & Weir, 1995b; Ray,Weir, Cullen, & Phillips, 1992) suggest that psychological factors play an important, if secondary role in CFS. In a factor-analytic study of 108 patients with CFS (Ray, Weir, Cullen, & Phillips, 1992), four symptom factors were found: emotional distress, fatigue, somatic symptoms, and cognitive difficulty. Although the symptom dimensions of fatigue, somatic symptoms, and cognitive difficulty were associated with general illness severity, emotional distress was not. The statistical independence of emotional states and perceived severity of illness could be one subjective basis on which patients deemphasize their pertinence and attribute the illness primarily to physical rather than psychological causes. Nevertheless, affect may contribute indirectly to the perception of illness severity to the extent that it is correlated with the other symptom dimensions (Ray, Weir, Cullen, & Phillips, 1992).

The hypothesized positive effect of pleasant mood on CFS has received preliminary empirical support. In a prospective study of 140 CFS patients (Ray et al.,1995b), positive events (which are presumably associated with pleasant emotions) were shown to predict improvements in fatigue, impairment, anxiety, and depression over a 1-year interval. Although these improvements did not reflect complete recovery, the study suggests that CFS and stress symptoms can be ameliorated to some degree with the generation of pleasant mood.

A coping skills–oriented cognitive–behavioral treatment study of CFS and primary depression (Friedberg & Krupp, 1994) suggests that emotional distress is more treatment-responsive than are CFS symptoms in high-functioning individuals. In this study, the subgroup of

CFS patients with the highest levels of comorbid depressive symptomatology showed the greatest reductions in depression, stress, and fatigue severity scores, although fatigue severity remained abnormally high. The coping skills based cognitive–behavioral intervention was far more effective for symptoms of stress and depression than it was for fatigue severity and its effect on functioning.

One plausible explanation for the lack of improvement in functioning in the Friedberg and Krupp (1994) study was the relatively high baseline activity level of the treatment sample. The majority of patients were working full- or half-time. Their reports of working to exhaustion were the primary reason that they rejected a therapist proposal for graded activity schedules. Perhaps, in high-functioning individuals with CFS, stress reduction is a more realistic goal than is substantial functional improvement. A comparison of coping skills and graded activity treatments in high-functioning CFS patients would provide an important empirical test of the illness reactivity model.

A review of psychological and behavioral studies of CFS (Friedberg & Jason, 1998) suggests that the illness reactivity model may better characterize high-functioning patients, whereas the symptom avoidance model may better explain the behavioral and symptomatic patterns of low-functioning patients with high levels of psychiatric morbidity.

Conversion Model

Finally, CFS has been described as a sociocultural phenomenon by Abbey and Garfinkel (1991b). These authors proposed that late-nineteenth-century neurasthenia, a CFS-like illness, and modern CFS have both occurred during social transformations in the role of women. More specifically, the rapidly changing role of women over the past two decades may have created an impossible set of cultural expectations to achieve in the workplace, to nurture a family, and to embrace social commitments. These cultural norms, although not consciously rejected by women, produce a debilitating conversion-like or psychophysiological illness that releases them from an array of burdensome obligations. Self-esteem is maintained by attribution of the (unconsciously) desired lifestyle change to medical illness (Powell, Dolan, & Wessely, 1990). The illness also allows female patients to receive the social and emotional support that they had presumably been lacking. Preliminary evidence in support of this model, as reviewed below, suggests that people with CFS (a) led overextended lifestyles, (b) were exposed to high numbers of pre-illness stressful events, and/or (c) received low levels of social support prior to becoming ill.

OVEREXTENDED LIFESTYLES

A qualitative study of 50 CFS patients (N. C. Ware & Kleinman, 1992) supports the above premise that individuals with CFS have been strongly committed to vocational and social accomplishment as well as caregiving in their families. In their study, the patients' narrative accounts of their illness were obtained. CFS sufferers described themselves as living overcommitted and overextended lives, which included a tendency to place the interests of others before their own. The data suggest that those who develop the illness may have adopted a social norm that featured exhaustion as a way of life. Paradoxically, 44% of the sample indicated that the illness was associated with positive realignment of life priorities such that they became more focused on personal goals of self-care and well-being rather than on the more external attachments to vocation and caregiving.

Without a comparison group of chronically ill non-CFS patients, it cannot be known if CFS-affected people are a distinct set of overachievers who were vulnerable to CFS or if individuals in any disabled, chronically ill group might describe themselves as high achievers in a society that encourages personal accomplishment. For example, in a study of Axis II disorders in patients with CFS or MS (Pepper et al., 1993), clinically significant elevations on the MCMI-II Compulsive Personality Disorder scale were found in 16% of the CFS patients and in 24% of the MS patients, a nonsignificant difference. Furthermore, in a comparison of patients with CFS and those with irritable bowel syndrome (Lewis, Cooper, & Bennett, 1994), no consistent differences were found between the two illness groups in the Type A behavior construct, which is associated with high-achievement behavior. However, both groups rated themselves as more "hard-driving" prior to illness onset than did healthy controls. Members of the CFS group also rated themselves as better listeners than did the other two groups, suggesting that CFS sufferers may manifest hard-driving behavior in setting high standards for interpersonal relationships. This conclusion is consistent with N. C. Ware and Kleinman's (1992) finding that CFS sufferers tend to be highly involved in helping others as well as doing other demanding activities. Another multigroup study (Van Houdenhove, Onghena, Neerinckx, & Hellin, 1995) also found that individuals with CFS reported hyperactive lifestyles premorbidly when compared with patients having chronic organ conditions or with other patients having various neurotic or dysthymic disturbances.

PRE-ILLNESS STRESS

Preliminary data for pre-illness stress in CFS patients have also been reported. In a comparative study of 134 CFS patients and 35 healthy controls (Salit, 1997), stressful events were found to be very common in the year preceding the onset of CFS (85%), but these occurred in only 6% of the controls. In the CFS study described earlier (Lewis et al., 1994), the authors suggested that the active problem-solving coping strategies preferred by individuals with CFS prior to illness onset may have been associated with increased stress. In contrast, certain emotion-focused coping strategies (e.g., tension reduction) eschewed by these CFS patients are more likely to be stress-reducing and restorative.

Further evidence suggests that pre-illness stress may be associated with CFS. In a controlled study, Stricklin, Sewell, and Austad (1990) found that in the 12 months prior to illness onset, participants with "epidemic neuromyasthenia," an acute fatiguing illness, experienced more loss-related life events than had healthy controls. In a subsequent case-controlled study of 20 individuals with CFS matched for age, sex, and race to healthy individuals (Dobbins, Natelson, Brassloff, Vrastal, & Sisto, 1995), participants reported significantly increased stress in the 5 years prior to their illness, compared with the healthy controls. Job stress, the death of someone close, and health-related stress were the most frequently endorsed stressful events. There was a dose–response relationship between the number of different sources of stress and the risk of illness.

Finally, in a small-sample retrospective study of prior trauma in CFS patients as compared with healthy controls (Schmaling & DiClementi, 1995), 77–78% of the two CFS groups reported sexual or physical abuse in childhood or adulthood, at least twice that reported by the control sample. The retrospective design of the aforementioned studies cannot rule out a possible reporting bias of CFS patients to inflate the frequency and magnitude of pre-illness stressors in an attempt to sustain self-perceptions as highly motivated individuals who have been struck by severe and debilitating chronic illness.

LOW LEVELS OF SOCIAL SUPPORT

Another important aspect of the conversion model is the hypothesized lack of social support experienced by patients prior to illness onset. In comparison to an irritable bowel syndrome group (Lewis et al., 1994), CFS participants reported low perceived social support in the 2 years prior to illness onset. Also, less social support has been associated with symptomatic relapse in a prospective study of the effects of a hurricane on CFS patients (Lutgendorf, Antoni, et al., 1995). These findings are consistent with a body of health outcome studies showing that low levels of social support are directly related to poorer physical and mental health (Berkman, 1995; Cohen & Herbert, 1996; Thoits, 1995).

Lack of social support has also been associated with higher serum cholesterol and uric acid levels and lower indices of immune function, including lymphocyte counts and nitrogen responses in healthy elderly people (Thomas, Goodwin, & Goodwin, 1985). It was hypothesized in this study that social support, defined as satisfying relationships with trusted individuals in whom the participants could confide, acted to reduce these physiological responses to stress. Similarly, an investigation of students' responses to the stress of a major course examination (Glaser, Kiecolt-Glaser, Speicher, & Holliday, 1985) revealed that higher levels of loneliness were associated with poorer immune function, that is, higher antibody titers to Epstein-Barr virus. A similar finding among married people with poor marital quality has also been reported (Kiecolt-Glaser, Fisher, Ogrocks, Stout, & Speicher, 1987).

On the other hand, adequate social support usually buffers the damaging effects of major life events and chronic strains on physical and mental health (Thoits, 1995). For instance, social relationships may lessen the effects of stress on neuroendocrine parameters (Seeman, Berkman, Blazer, & Rowe, 1994) and improve immune function in spouses of patients with cancer (Cohen & Herbert, 1996). In a study of neuroendocrine function and social support (Seeman et al., 1994), social relations—especially the generality of emotional support—was related to healthier urinary levels of epinephrine, norepinephrine, and cortisol among older high-functioning men and women.

CONCLUSIONS

Although some aspects of the conversion model are supported by the previously cited retrospective reports and correlational evidence, a longitudinal study following healthy people who become ill would be necessary to determine the nature of the relationship between the postulated pre-illness stressors and subsequent illness. However, the conversion model neglects to consider the interaction between stress variables, symptom-producing immune defects, and neuroendocrine abnormalities in the pathogenesis of the illness. A weaker reconceptualization of the conversion model, based on current evidence, might be stated as follows: Given some evidence for impaired immune function (Blondel-Hill & Shafran, 1993) and cortisol deficits (Demitrack et al., 1991) in CFS, the co-occurrence of unhealthy psychosocial influences, such as pre-illness stress or inadequate social support, may increase vulnerability to the illness.

Psychoneuroimmunology and CFS

It is unclear which combination of biological and psychiatric factors are causing and maintaining CFS. Given this uncertainty, a psychoneuroimmunology model might provide health care professionals with a heuristic framework for understanding this disease syndrome. Psychoneuroimmunologists propose that the nervous, endocrine, and immune systems are in constant communication with each other (Kiecolt-Glaser & Glaser, 1989). In the mid-1970s, Ader and Cohen's (1975) pioneering work indicated that the immune system can be conditioned, suggesting that our thoughts and surroundings can cue immune enhancement or suppression. Reductions in the number of disease-fighting immune cells occur under conditions of stress, depression, loss of control, learned helplessness, high anxiety, bereavement, loneliness, or inhibited high power motivation (Kiecolt-Glaser, Garner, Speicher, Penn, & Glaser, 1984).

According to Kaplan (1991), a variety of factors might influence immunosuppression, including dysphoric responses (e.g., depressive affect, unhappiness, anxiety), immunosuppressive behaviors (e.g., dietary patterns, sleep habits, licit and illicit drug use), adverse life experiences (e.g., ongoing strains in interpersonal relationships), and preexisting vulnerabilities (e.g., the absence of interpersonal resources and coping patterns to forestall the impact of negative life experiences). Many studies have provided some support for components of this theory (e.g., D. M. Clark, 1986; Pennebaker & Beall, 1986). These theoretical ideas might have important implications for understanding CFS. The data presented below examine (a) the interactions between personality traits and coping and (b) biologic processes within the framework of psychoneuroimmunology.

PERSONALITY TRAITS AND COPING

Personality tendencies may have a significant influence on the likelihood of illness. Repressors, who are unaware of negative feelings, will deny feeling anxiety when stressed, but they show large increases in physical signs of overstimulation (e.g., heart rate, muscle tension; Jamner & Schwartz, 1986). Constant stimulation of the sympathetic nervous system can result in a flood of stress hormones (e.g., adrenaline), which may increase the risk of heart disease and also suppress the immune system. Repressors may inhibit the perception of anxiety, anger, and sadness by synthesizing high levels of endorphins, which are natural painkillers that dull experiences of discomfort. Thus, repressors can function in painful jobs or family relationships by using increasing doses of natural "painkillers" (endorphins) to repress psychic wounds. This cycle of emotional pain and repression can ultimately lead to psychological collapse or physical illness (Jamner & Schwartz, 1986).

The tendency to ignore or repress bodily sensations and negative emotions is related to weaker immune functions, whereas those who are more aware of their body–mind states and express their feelings have stronger immune functions (Jamner, Schwartz, & Leigh, 1988). Dreher (1995) has summarized research suggesting that repressive coping in patients is correlated with a variety of infectious diseases as well as immune-related illnesses such as lupus, allergies, asthma, and cancer. A coping strategy of denial, a form of repression, has been associated with greater illness burdens in CFS (Antoni et al., 1994).

Whereas inhibition of thoughts and feelings is linked to internal stress, expression of memories and feelings associated with traumas allows the nervous system to relax, resulting in improvements in immune function and the ability to resist disease (Pennebaker, Kiecolt-Glaser, & Glaser, 1988). However, caution needs to be exercised in applying these findings more generally to people with CFS. S. K. Johnson, DeLuca, and Natelson (1996c) found that the most prevalent personality dimensions in CFS patients are in the highly emotional cluster, as opposed to the more repressive, nondisclosing styles.

The need for power, and the satisfaction or frustration of that need, may also be considered in a discussion of psychoneuroimmunological factors. Strong power needs are healthy when they are expressed apppropriately and balanced with a value for relationships (McClelland, Floor, Davidson, & Saron, 1980). However, people with inhibited power motives tend to be angry and argumentative and live in a constant state of tension. With the wish for mastery frustrated, the resulting anger and anxiety cause stress hormones to remain at high levels, overstimulating the heart and reducing the strength of the immune system (McClelland et al., 1980). The weakened immune function in these individuals increases their susceptibility to infections. A strong need for power combined with a weaker need for affiliation results in increased vulnerability to many types of illness, especially upper respiratory infections. On the other hand, those who pursue relationships without excessive anxiety, and who value social relationships over power, suffer fewer bouts of illness (McClelland et al., 1980).

Other psychological traits also have important implications for the immune system. For example, hardiness is composed of three distinct but interconnected qualities: commitment, control, and challenge. Kobasa, Maddi, Puccetti, and Zola (1985) found that executives who possessed these personality traits, received adequate social support, and did regular exercise showed a likelihood of illness of only 8%, whereas those without these resources had a likelihood of illness of 92%.

Studies of AIDS patients indicate that certain personality traits have survival value. In a recent summary of the research, Dreher (1995) indicated that AIDS patients with a greater sense of personal control have a stronger immune system and live longer. In addition to a sense of control, assertiveness and a fighting spirit seem to be key factors among long-term AIDS survivors (Solomon, Temoshok, O'Leary, & Zich, 1987) and may prevent other diseases of weakened immunity.

Coping and mood may also be affected by the severity of intrusive symptoms. Exacerbation of symptoms in CFS may trigger maladaptive appraisals and coping strategies, which may prolong symptomatic episodes via affective, neuroendocrine, and immunologic pathways (Antoni et al., 1994). In addition, changes in mood, fatigue, and malaise are commonly associated with infectio n (Ray, 1991). Depression and anxiety can be a psychological reaction to a serious illness, as is common in patients with cancer and heart disease. Ray (1991) believes that depressive reactions to prolonged illness, such as CFS, may be better conceptualized as demoralization rather than psychiatric illness, particularly in ambiguous illnesses where patients have difficulty gaining medical recognition.

BIOLOGIC FACTORS

The psychoneuroimmunology concepts summarized below may be difficult to understand, particularly for those whose biological knowledge is less extensive. However, these physiologic processes are important because they provide researchers with critical leads to better understand the complex interactive processes that underlie CFS.

A number of studies suggest that CFS and associated stress symptoms may be caused in part by disruptions in immune and neurological function. Because the onset of CFS is often linked with recent viral infection or other illness in the patient's biological systems, a study of the syndrome's neuroimmunological aspects might appropriately begin with a look at how the brain tends to adapt to infection. After a viral infection, the brain is exposed to high levels of various (fatigue-related) cytokines, which are naturally occurring hormones produced in the course of an immunological response to infection. Activation by macrophages (immune system cells that ingest dead tissues and cellular debris) in response to a virus or bacterium produces a release of the cytokine interleukin 1 (IL-1). IL-1 causes an alteration in electrical activity of the brain as well as behavioral changes, (e.g., decreases in activity or social interaction; somnolence). These behavioral reactions reduce unnecessary energy expenditures so that available energy stores can be used to fight the infection (Maier, Watkins, & Fleshner, 1994).

Cytokines such as IL-1 could induce a state of chronic immune activation, which would lead to a depletion of the stress hormone axis, a condition that has been associated with CFS (Saphier, 1994). Some individuals might be at higher risk for developing such chronic activation, due to genetic vulnerabilities or to constitutional, psychological, or environmental factors. For instance, environmental factors might play a role in the etiology of CFS, as people with CFS have significantly higher levels of chlorinated hydrocarbons in their urinary metabolites than do control participants (Dunstan et al., 1995).

Another area of neurological research that has implications for understanding CFS involves chronic activation of the sympathetic nervous system. Girdano, Everly, and Dusek (1990) have summarized research indicating that increased sympathetic tone may be related to a wide variety of disorders, including ventricular fibrillation in the absence of coronary heart disease, essential hypertension, coronary artery disease, migraine headache, Raynaud's disease, and irritable bowel syndrome. Gellhorn (1970) and Gellhorn and Keily (1972) have further postulated that under prolonged stimulation of the limbic-hypothalamic-pituitary axis, a lowered threshold for sympathetic activation can occur. In other words, low levels of stimulation that would not adversely affect a healthy person can elicit prolonged high levels of arousal in individuals with the above cited disorders. This high level of sympathetic tone is implicated in many disorders of the immune system and may occur in CFS. The process leading to increased sympathetic tone is called *tuning*.

Once the sympathetic nervous system is tuned or "charged," either by high-intensity stimulation or by chronically repeated low-intensity stimulation, it may sustain a high level of arousal (Gellhorn, 1968). Girdano et al. (1990) suggested that this excessive arousal can lead to an increase in the number of dendrites in the limbic system, which may further increase limbic stimulation. Overall, the limbic system is growing more excitatory postsynaptic receptors while its inhibitory presynaptic receptors are decreasing. As inhibition of neuronal firing is decreased and excitation is increased, the brain may become hypersensitive to stress due to a decreased threshold for neuronal excitability.

Paul Cheney, a prominent scientist-clinician in the field of CFS, supports this tuning hypothesis (Carpman, 1995; Zivin & Choi, 1991). Cheney hypothesizes that people with CFS have excitatory neurotoxicity, explained as follows: Two receptors, residing on the cell surface membranes of neurons, are designated gamma-aminobutyric acid (GABA), which inhibit neuronal firing, and N-methyl-D-aspartate (NMDA), which excite neuronal firing. These functions of the GABA and NMDA receptors are normally balanced, but after an injury, the

NMDA receptors fire more than do the GABA receptors. This imbalance scrambles information processing, puts stress on the neuron, and, if severe enough, will kill the neuron. The clinical observations of Cheney in treating hundreds of patients with CFS suggest that almost every drug that down-regulates NMDA receptor firing (e.g., benzodiazipine therapy, magnesium, Nimotop, melatonin, calcium channel blockers), and presumably restores the GABA–NMDA balance, has been helpful for people with CFS (Carpman, 1995).

The aforementioned physiological concepts of CFS reactivity are endorsed by Goldstein (1990), who also believes that in a person with CFS, the brain has become hypersensitive to stress. Through *kindling*, a type of sensitization, which, like tuning, causes a decreased threshold for neuronal excitability, a neuron might begin to fire uncontrollably in reaction to one or more minor stimuli. In support of the kindling theory, Brouwer and Packer (1994) have conducted research indicating that people with CFS might have "unstable cortical excitability associated with sustained muscle activity resulting in varied magnitudes of descending volleys" (p. 1212). If individuals with this syndrome have such chronic activation of the central nervous system, then one of the key features of effective treatments might be to decrease excitatory neurotoxicity.

Other evidence also supports the notion of a primary neuronal defect. The hypothesis that CFS involves a state of reduced central sympathetic drive via increased firing of the locus coeruleus has received support from two studies of pharmacological intervention. Natelson et al. (1996) reported that low-dose treatment with a monamine oxidase inhibitor produced a significant pattern of improvement with CFS patients. Other research by Snorrason, Geirsson, and Stefansson (1996) found that 70% of CFS patients reported at least a 30% improvement when treated with galanthamine hydrobromide, which is a selective inhibitor of acetycholinesterase. Also, galanthamine increases plasma levels of cortisol. In general, these drugs help to reduce locus coeruleus firing and increase central sympathetic neurotransmission to sensitized receptors, a process that produces a restorative neural desensitization. These findings point to a cholinergic deficit as a key feature of CFS.

MULTIPLE PATHWAYS, MULTIVARIATE ILLNESS

There might be various pathways into the neurobiologic disregulations described above, with a viral infection representing just one possible route. This might be the reason why some people with CFS had viral infections, while others had other medical illnesses, before they developed CFS (Wessely et al., 1995). In addition, it is possible that viral infection can occur in the absence of inflammation; in these cases, the virus evades the host immune system and allows the functions of the cell to continue. For example, there is evidence of persistent cytomegalovirus infection in the pancreatic cells of people with diabetes (Wessely, 1993). Thus, for some individuals, the virus could be the primary cause of later onset CFS, but the absence of initial viral symptoms would make the infected person unaware that he or she was sick.

Another possible illness pathway is the disruption in circadian rhythmicity, recently found in CFS patients (Williams et al., 1996). Such a disruption may cause fatigue and cognitive symptoms, results similar to the reactions of healthy people who are kept awake during their habitual sleep period. Evidence for a dissociation of circadian rhythms in people with CFS has been reported by Williams et al. (1996): Whereas body temperature and melatonin secretion were significantly correlated in healthy controls, no significant correlation was found in patients with CFS.

Rather than conceptualizing CFS as an illness of solely the body or the mind, psychoneuroimmunology provides a transactional model, which suggests that complex interactions between multiple biological and psychological factors influence the onset of CFS and subsequent pathways to further illness or recovery.

THE PROBLEM OF HETEROGENEITY IN CFS

It is probable that different types of illnesses are contained within the CFS construct, which complicates the task of identifying patient commonalities within the diagnosis. For example, in one study (Friedberg, McKenzie, Dechene, & Fontanetta, 1994), those patients who improved over time had significantly more severe CFS symptoms during the first year of their illness. In another study, Hickie et al. (1995) found two subsets within their CFS samples: 73% were clustered in a heterogeneous group with limited fatigue and neuropsychiatric symptoms, and moderate disability; the remaining 27% had clinical characteristics of somatoform disorders, including numerous somatic and psychological symptoms, more illness behavior, and severe psychological morbidity. Similarly, S. K. Johnson et al. (1996c) have found that the 34% of their CFS sample with a current depressive diagnosis accounted for most of the personality pathology, which supports the utility of categorizing CFS patients according to psychiatric diagnosis.

An immunomodulatory treatment of CFS also points to the importance of subgrouping analyses. See and Tilles (1996) found that alpha interferon treatment significantly improved quality of life scores only for those with NK cell dysfunction, suggesting that this subgroup of CFS patients benefited from the increased cytokine production, triggered by the interferon-stimulated NK cells. This process may have led to restoration of normal immune function.

Even the construct of fatigue needs to be better differentiated into various dimensions (e.g., postexercise symptoms, flare-up symptoms, remission symptoms, allergy fatigue; Dechene, Friedberg, McKenzie, & Fontanetta, 1994). Until better differentiated subgroups are developed, it will be exceedingly difficult to identify characteristics that are common for all people with the diagnosis of CFS.

The four models of CFS, presented at the beginning of the chapter, may also reflect the heterogeneity of the illness. Qualitatively different subgroups may be best explained by different models. For instance, some low-functioning patients may be more likely to fear and avoid symptom flare-ups, consistent with the symptom avoidance model, whereas high-functioning CFS patients who show no evidence of fearful avoidance may be better understood within the illness reactivity model. Thus, it seems likely that each model will evolve in its explanatory power as subgroup analysis and classification progresses, based on new biological, psychiatric, and psychosocial evidence for pathogenetic factors in CFS.

II | ASSESSMENT

Measurement of CFS Symptoms | 4

Because CFS, as currently defined, is a multidimensional behavioral construct rather than a precisely delineated disease entity, sophisticated behavioral assessment is crucial. In particular, we believe that the full spectrum of symptom severity must be assessed, rather than the mere presence or absence of symptoms. In this chapter, we emphasize the importance of a better-differentiated system for collecting data on CFS symptoms that goes beyond the simple binary system used with the case definition. Such a system can help clinicians and investigators gain a greater appreciation of the fluctuating nature of this illness, the intrapersonal variability of symptoms, and the debilitation associated with this chronic condition. We suggest specific guidelines to assess symptom severity in order to improve diagnostic accuracy and refine the current case definition. We also show why it is important to collect data over time and to observe how fatigue is related to activity levels when evaluating fatigue in the CFS patient.

In the last section of the chapter, we explain how the use of actigraphs can provide more accurate, fine-grained assessment and evaluation of treatment programs. Finally, a series of case studies show clinicians and researchers the benefits of using richer, more precise measurements to gather data on symptoms and activity patterns of CFS patients.

Limitations of Binary Classification: The Risk of Misdiagnosis

CFS is currently defined by the presence of a constellation of psychological, neuropsychological, and physical symptoms that accompany severe levels of fatigue. The symptom criteria for the eight minor symptoms (e.g., sore throat, muscle pain), described in chapter 1, play a pivotal role in the assessment and diagnosis of this syndrome. Yet despite the importance of these symptoms in defining CFS, current approaches to charting and assessing symptoms rely on data collected at only one time point, and only the presence or absence (binary classification) of symptoms is assessed (with the exception of Jason, Holden, Taylor, & Melrose, 1995; Jason & Taylor, 1994; and Wood, Magnello, & Sharpe, 1992).

The binary nature of the definition of CFS contributes to wide variations in assessment findings among studies of CFS (Bates et al., 1994). For example, Jason, Taylor, et al. (1995) found, in a recent epidemiology study, that the scoring of only the occurrence or nonoccurrence CFS symptoms (Fukuda et al., 1994) resulted in 2% of the participants being identified as (possibly) having CFS. Yet, after participants completed a medical workup, it was found that only .2% of the sample actually had CFS (Jason, Taylor, et al., 1995). In another study using a binary screening scale for CFS definitional symptoms (Jason, Ropacki, et al., 1997), four groups were assessed: CFS, lupus, MS, and a healthy control group. If self-reported symptoms alone had been used to differentiate these samples, 100% of the CFS group would have been identified with CFS—but 27% of the MS group and 73% of the lupus group would also have met the Fukuda et al. (1994) definition for CFS. In a related finding (Dechene et al., 1994), 15% of a group of 179 healthy middle-aged people met criteria for CFS, based on the self-reported presence or absence of each definitional symptom.

These findings demonstrate the potential for misdiagnosis of CFS if only broad measures, limited to the occurrence or nonoccurrence of specific symptoms, are used. Alternatively, more precise symptom measures may lead to greater diagnostic accuracy. If the symptoms identified by Fukuda et al. (1994) were better differentiated (e.g., severity ratings on a 100-point scale), health care professionals would have a greater ability to distinguish the symptoms of CFS from those of other fatiguing illnesses.

In addition to obscuring the variability that people with CFS experience in their symptomatology, current binary rating scales also provide limited information about the high interpersonal variability of this illness. For example, two individuals may both indicate the presence of a particular symptom; however, for one person the severity of the symptom may be mild, while for the other it might be severe (Jason, Holden, et al., 1995).

The findings of a large sample ($N = 565$) descriptive study (Hickie et al., 1995) underscore the value of measuring symptom severity when assessing individuals with CFS. This sample of patients diagnosed with CFS were clinically and statistically divided into two subgroups according to their clinical symptomatology. Seventy-three percent of the participants were classified into a group that had moderate disability, limited fatigue, and neuropsychological symptoms. The remaining patients reported greater disability, more severe symptoms, a much higher number of atypical CFS symptoms, and in general showed the clinical characteristics of a somatoform disorder. Thus, for this large sample of patients with CFS, the symptom profile was not unimodal. Through observation of the severity and number of symptoms, meaningful differences were found between the two subgroups on most clinical markers of CFS (Hickie et al., 1995).

Case Studies Using Symptom Severity Ratings

In addition to symptom ratings, assessing symptoms at more than one time point will also improve diagnostic accuracy and document illness fluctuations. Jason and Taylor (1994) devised a series of simple-to-use rating scales to profile CFS symptoms and show changes in symptoms over time. For one female patient with CFS, symptoms were rated from 0 = *no problem* to 10 = *severe problem*. Figure 4.1 shows the ratings at one time-period during the participant's worst month *(A)*, and at a follow-up one and a half years later, when many of the worst symptoms had subsided *(B)*. This individual was not working during the first assessment and was working on a part-time basis at follow-up. At both assessments, the participant had a greater than 50% reduction in both energy level and activity level. The visual analysis provides a stark depiction of the severity of her symptoms. In addition, the charting of symptoms at different time points reveals a slow pattern of progress; this type of recovery process has been described by D.S. Bell (1991).

A subsequent study (Jason, King, Frankenberry, Jordan, & Tryon, 1998) refined the Jason and Taylor (1994) measurement system and further demonstrated the advantages of such an approach in the assessment of one case of CFS and one healthy control participant.

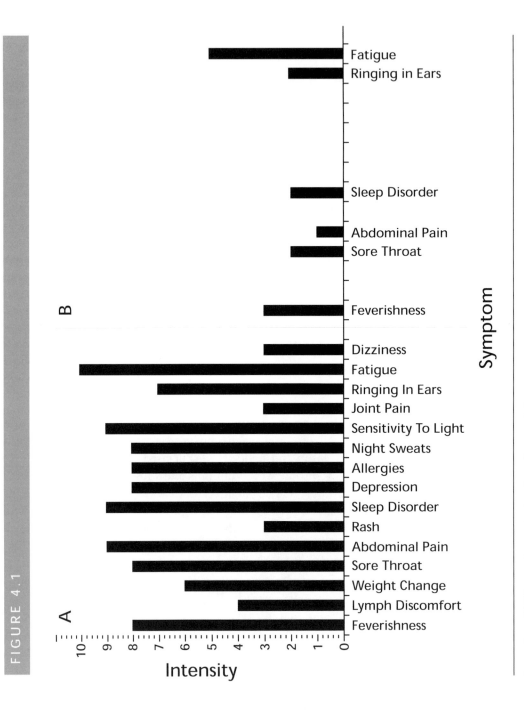

Intensity of CFS symptoms during two time points.

These individuals completed a CFS Symptom Rating Form (see Appendix C) on which they rated levels of fatigue, CFS definitional symptoms, and other somatic and cognitive symptoms frequently experienced by people with CFS (D.S. Bell, 1991; Holmes, Kaplan, Gantz, et al., 1988). Symptoms were rated on a 100-point scale, with 0 = *no fatigue, pain,* etc. and 100 = *severe fatigue, pain,* etc. The participants were asked to rate retrospectively the symptoms they experienced during the worst period of their illness and then to rate current symptoms on the day of assessment.

The rated somatic symptoms (other than CFS definitional symptoms) included racing heart, chest pain, shortness of breath, upset stomach, weight change, dizziness, ringing in the ears, sweating hands, night sweats, tense muscles, chills or shivering, hot or cold spells, feverish feeling, lowered temperature, tingling feeling, paralysis, blurred vision, light sensitivity, blind spots, eye pain, rash, and allergies. The rated cognitive symptoms included slowness of thought, absent-mindedness, confusion, reasoning difficulties, forgetting thoughts, difficulty choosing words, difficulty concentrating, difficulty understanding, and slowed reactions. A more detailed presentation of these data may be found in Jason, King, et al. (1998).

The healthy control participant in this study was a 51-year-old White male teacher who was not suffering from CFS or any other chronic illnesses. Nevertheless, he had experienced a number of the CFS definitional symptoms. In fact, when standard assessment procedures (i.e., binary classification) were used, his symptom reports nearly met criteria for CFS (presence of fatigue and three minor symptoms). However, his symptom severity ratings clarified the nature of his condition. His fatigue and all three of his minor symptoms were rated as being quite mild (5 on the 100-point scale) and nondisabling. Had data been collected only on symptom occurrence and not on symptom severity, his symptom profile would have shown many of the characteristics of a person with CFS. Moreover, his symptoms might have been considered suggestive of serious or chronic illness.

In contrast to this healthy control participant, Lois, a 47-year-old retired White woman, developed CFS 5½ years ago. It began with an infection contracted in the hospital following a surgical procedure. During the first 3 years of her illness, Lois was completely "wiped out" and estimated that her capacity to function was impaired by 95%. In the past 2½ years, she has experienced some symptom relief and now rates her level of impairment at 70%. Figure 4.2 presents a comparison of Lois's severity ratings for the CFS definitional symptoms during the worst period of her illness, approximately 5½ years ago, and on the day of data collection. During the worst period of her illness (95%

FIGURE 4.2

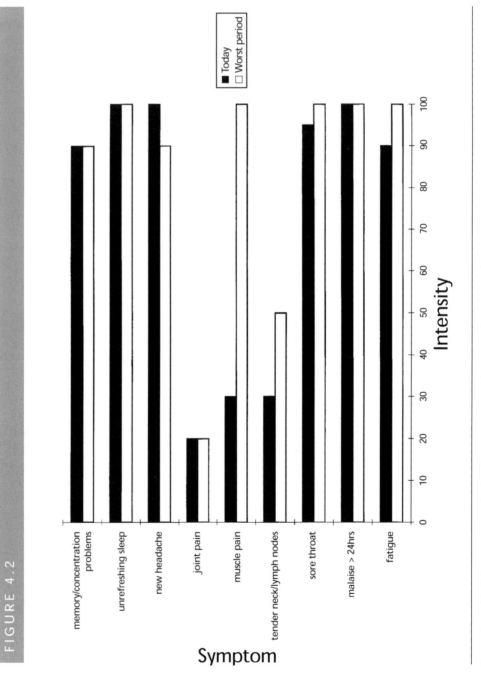

Intensity of Lois's symptoms during her worst time (about 5½ years ago) and at a recent assessment.

impaired function), she rated her CFS definitional symptoms as extremely severe. At the time of data collection, when she reported 70% overall impairment, a number of her CFS definitional symptoms were rated as less severe. Figure 4.2 shows the modest symptomatic improvements Lois experienced for CFS definitional symptoms.

The case of Lois illustrates the importance of charting in the assessment of illness severity over time. She reported only slight reductions in CFS definitional symptoms despite a moderate improvement in functioning. The charting clearly quantified these changes and indicated that the patient continued to be quite ill.

In contrast to this individual with CFS, the healthy control participant's symptoms were extremely mild. The assessment of symptom severity rather than symptom occurrence alone facilitated an accurate differential diagnosis for both the healthy participant and the individual with CFS.

Clinical Implications of Symptom Charting

We have observed marked improvements over time with some CFS patients, although their ongoing symptoms and functional limitations still meet criteria for the diagnosis of CFS. Health care providers and caregivers cannot assume that marked reductions in symptomatology are indicative of full recovery. When significant improvements are obtained and patients feel better, many of these individuals are still impaired considerably by CFS and do not view themselves as "recovered." Symptom charting can confirm the presence of ongoing illness.

It is clear from the case studies presented in this book that CFS is a highly individualized illness. Different patients present distinct clinical pictures of symptomatology and severity. Had quantitative data not been collected on symptom severity through the use of rating scales for the patient just described (Lois), such critical differences would have gone unrecognized. Furthermore, by charting this data and obtaining symptom patterns, the clinician can gain valuable feedback regarding the impact of patients' coping strategies on their health status. Such information can assist in the successful management and treatment of CFS. For example, symptoms rated "very problematic" might be identified and treated before other symptoms with less severe ratings. Given the many symptoms of this complex illness and the variable nature of its symptomatology, approaches that provide quantitative data over time are needed to improve our understanding of the illness.

Standardized Symptom Measurement and the Case Definition

It is hoped that future definitions of CFS will include specific guidelines pertaining to the importance of symptom severity in the diagnostic procedure. Health care professionals may need a standardized procedure to determine if a particular symptom is severe enough to qualify as one of the symptoms required for the diagnosis of CFS. Currently there are no guidelines for physicians to evaluate symptom severity when using the diagnostic criteria. If CFS is to be diagnosed reliably across health care professions, cutoffs—points at which symptoms are not considered to be severe enough to meet the case definition for CFS—may be needed to lend precision to the diagnostic procedure.

Without such standardization, the sample of individuals diagnosed with CFS is likely to vary, not necessarily as a function of etiological factors alone, but rather as a function of assessment procedures as well. If health care professionals are to improve their understanding of the symptom dimensions of this disease and identify clinically important subtypes of patients with CFS, then the current U.S. case definition will require empirically guided revisions.

Problems in Fatigue Assessment

One of the more vexing problems in the assessment process involves the selection of adequate measures of perceived fatigue and energy (D.S. Bell, 1991). Barofsky and Legro (1991) reviewed a number of single-item and multiple-item scales designed to measure degree of fatigue (see also chap. 5 in this book). For example, Krupp, La Rocca, Muir-Nash, & Steinberg, (1989) used a seven-point Fatigue Severity Scale (1 = *no fatigue*, 7 = *fatigue*) to measure the relationship between fatigue and functioning. This easy-to-administer instrument has been included in assessments of CFS (Krupp et al., 1991). Such scales typically have been used to provide a symptom severity estimate for a single time point.

An alternative assessment strategy has been offered by Wood et al. (1992), who collected data on energy levels over time with a sample of CFS patients. This type of ongoing assessment seems critical in order to understand symptoms that often appear and disappear for sometimes brief and sometimes protracted periods. In this study, patients with CFS rated their physical and mental energy and their positive and negative affect six times daily for 7 days. Although ratings of these subjective states yielded insights into daily patterns of perceived energy and affect, other important variables, including activity levels and other symptoms, were not rated. Fatigue might best be understood in its relationship to activity level because some CFS-afflicted individuals may experience little fatigue if they restrict their activities, whereas others may experience extreme fatigue with only minor or moderate activity.

Case Studies With Hourly Fatigue and Stress Monitoring

Because fatigue levels constitute such a prominent and defining feature of CFS, a behavioral approach using time-series methods might be useful in describing and understanding fatigue patterns in CFS. The following case studies illustrate such an approach for patients with CFS (Jason, Holden, et al., 1995).

Peter had been diagnosed with CFS by two independent physicians. For 2 consecutive days, starting at 6:00 a.m. and lasting until 6:00 p.m., data were collected each hour for two of his primary symptoms: feverishness (0 = *normal*, 10 = *severe problem*) and fatigue (0 = *normal*, 10 = *severe problem*). During each hourly period, the slight presence or definite presence of the following four moods was also recorded: anger, obsessiveness, calm, and happiness. In addition, any uplifts (desirable events; 1 = *minor*, 2 = *moderate*, 3 = *extreme*) or hassles (undesirable events; 1 = *minor*, 2 = *moderate*, 3 = *extreme*) were rated. Finally, activity level (1 = *practically none*, 10 = *excessive*), which was defined as subjectively rated energy expenditure for walking, working, thinking, and so on, was recorded hourly. Figure 4.3 presents Peter's data on the symptom of fatigue and activity level, starting hourly at 6:00 a.m.

It is clear that, as activity level increased—particularly in the morning—the intensity of the primary symptom of fatigue increased as well. Hassles and obsessions also occurred in the morning while the participant was at work. When activities decreased and the participant rested or relaxed at home, the symptoms tended to decrease. Peter usually felt stronger in the morning, but after 3 hours of work at the office, symptoms of fatigue and fever rose to moderate levels and then decreased rapidly after resting. Yet this symptom pattern represented

FIGURE 4.3

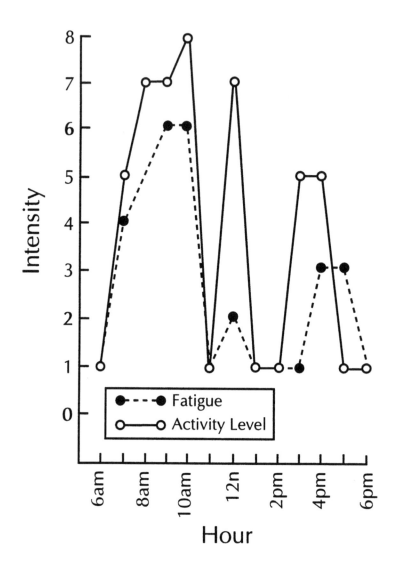

Hourly data for intensity of Peter's symptom of fatigue and activity level.

FIGURE 4.4

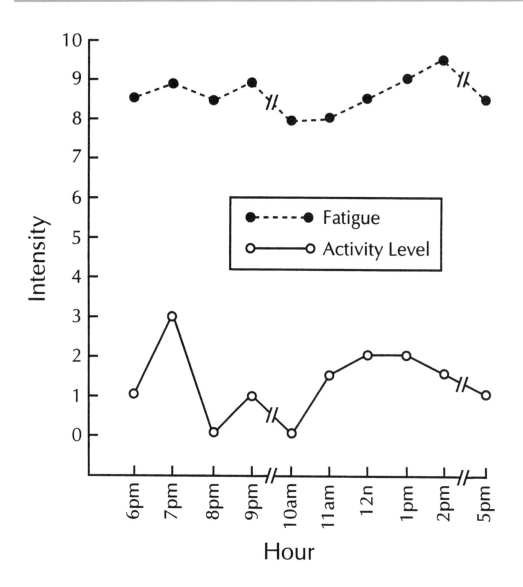

Hourly data for intensity of Mary's fatigue and activity level.

an improvement. Only 1 year earlier, Peter had experienced higher fatigue levels and was unable to do any work.

A different behavioral pattern is illustrated in a second case, that of Mary, who was also diagnosed with CFS by two physicians. She slept about 15 hours per day, and her daily activity consisted of walking around the house or completing a necessary errand.

Activity level, defined as energy expenditure for sitting, driving, thinking, and so forth, was rated in comparison with Mary's typical premorbid activity level (0 = *at premorbid level,* 10 = *substantially different from premorbid level*). Her primary symptoms, fatigue and sore throat, were rated on a 10-point severity scale (0 = *none,* 10 = *severe*). The types of moods rated were labeled "calm," "mild anxiety," and "mild depression." Data were not available for the hours between 9:00 p.m. and 10:00 a.m., and again for the hours between 2:00 and 5:00 p.m., because the participant slept during these periods. Figure 4.4 charts the hourly changes that occurred during one 24-hour period for fatigue and activity level. The graph shows that Mary's symptoms were rated as severe at all time points, even though activity level was rather low.

In sum, Peter's behavioral patterning was very distinct from that recorded by Mary. Fatigue for Peter fluctuated dramatically over time and was associated with activity level and mood. In contrast, Mary's fatigue levels were consistently high, although a modest positive relationship appeared between activity and fatigue.

A recent pilot study (Jason, King, Tryon, Frankenberry, & Jordan, 1997) collected behavioral data to show some of the benefits that can be derived from monitoring both hourly and daily symptoms. On a 100-point scale, one participant with CFS was asked to rate perceived energy (0 = *no energy;* 100 = *abundant energy,* similar to energy levels when completely well) and mental and physical exertion, also on a 100-point scale. Modeling with time-series regression revealed several statistically significant correlates of fatigue, both within and between days. In both analyses, perceived energy was negatively related to fatigue, whereas physical and mental exertion were positively related to fatigue.

Collection of time-series data may produce the clinical data needed to revise and refine the Fukuda et al. (1994) definition of CFS. For instance, the definition stipulates that the fatigue (in CFS) is not the result of ongoing exertion; however, as mentioned earlier, some patients may experience a major increase in fatigue after minimal exertion. A revised definition might incorporate an in vivo activity and fatigue assessment rather than assume that fatigue is a static feature of CFS. In general, the important interrelationships between fatigue symptoms, energy levels, activity, mood, and stress need to be addressed and clarified in the case definition.

Next, we ask, "Are perceived energy, fatigue, and exertion ratings related to actual behavior?" We now consider this issue.

Actigraphy

A front-page article by Azar (1997) in the *APA Monitor* reported on a National Institutes of Health (NIH) conference held to discuss problems with self-report data. According to the article, self-report data may lead to erroneous research results more often than was previously thought. However, self-report format is unavoidable for some variables such as fatigue, which is a complex psychophysiological state that cannot as yet be measured otherwise. This is clearly not the case, however, for activity for which objective instrumented measurements are available and constitute a gold standard (Tryon, 1991). Tryon and Williams (1996) have described a new computerized actigraph capable of measuring the intensity of activity and recording such values every minute of the day and night for 22 consecutive days. This technology for obtaining objective longitudinal activity measurements while the participant behaves in his or her natural environment can and should be used to examine closely the relationships between behavior and the symptoms of fatigue.

Pilot data have recently been collected on the actigraph for two CFS participants over a period of 2 to 3 weeks (Jason, King, et al., 1998). The actigraph measurement showed that the individuals with CFS had far fewer episodes of intense physical activity in comparison with a healthy control participant. More specifically, the healthy participant exhibited high levels of activity during the day (5,000–6,000 units) and low levels at night, whereas the participants with CFS did not show the high spiking of daytime activity. Additional actigraph data were significantly related to self-reported indices of expended energy and physical and mental exertion (Jason, Tryon, Frankenberry, & King, 1997). Actigraphy data for the healthy control participant and one of the participants with CFS are presented in Figures 4.5 and 4.6, respectively.

Another recent study (Fry & Martin, 1996) examined measures of activity for children with CFS and for healthy controls. When an objective measure of activity (Gaehwiler Activity Monitor) averaged over a 3-day period was analyzed, there were no significant differences between the two groups. Looking at overall daily levels of activity could be misleading, however, as it is the *pattern* of activity that may be most important in differentiating people with CFS from controls.

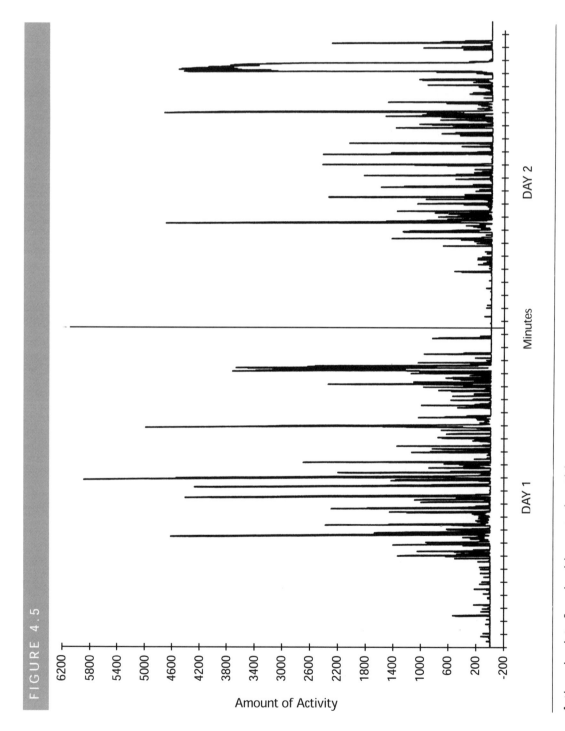

FIGURE 4.5

Actigraphy data for a healthy control participant.

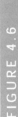

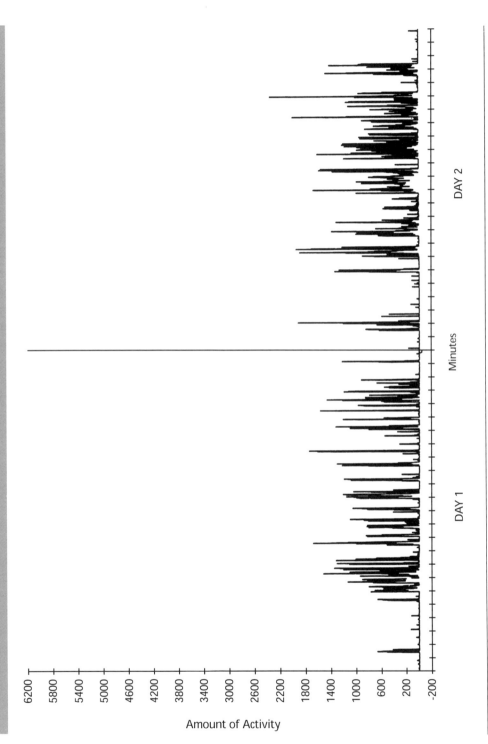

FIGURE 4.6

Actigraphy data for a person with CFS.

On the other hand, child and parent ratings of activity were significantly greater for the healthy controls. For the CFS group, the children's desired level of activity was significantly higher than their expected level of activity in the future, whereas the healthy children showed no significant difference between the desired and expected levels of activity.

The authors believed that the discrepancy between expectation and desire may play a role in maintaining the illness. If children with CFS have desired goals that are unattainable, they may avoid the challenge and thus, the inevitable disappointment. An alternative explanation of the findings would be that the children with CFS might desire to be more active, but based on current health problems, they are not optimistic about being more active and healthy in the future.

Summary

This chapter argues against the current binary system of symptom evaluation to define CFS. Rather than recording the mere presence or absence of particular symptoms, we have cited in vivo data that show how the assessment of symptom severity over multiple time points will improve our understanding of the wide variability of symptoms in CFS patients. Case studies that collected time-series data also revealed clinically meaningful relationships between fatigue and activity level that may have important implications for defining CFS. Such fine-grained methods of assessment will also provide a better understanding of the experiences of patients with this illness. Finally, the recommendations in this chapter may be useful to systematically evaluate treatment programs geared toward people with CFS.

Fatigue Rating Scales 5

uscio (1921) concluded in his analysis of fatigue and its measurement that the empirically vague term *fatigue* should "be absolutely banished from scientific discussion, and consequently that attempts to obtain a fatigue test be abandoned" (p. 31). As in 1921, the term *fatigue* continues to elude precise definition or objective measurement in the research literature (Barofsky & Legro, 1991). Although fatigue is a nonspecific symptom occurring in most physical illnesses and many psychiatric disorders, it has not been differentiated by illness or defined by its behavioral and situational contexts. Thus, in CFS, fatigue may be related to physical exertion, emotional stress, pain, sleep disturbance, depression, or the poorly understood causal mechanisms of the illness (Barofsky & Legro, 1991).

An early proposal for a fatigue rating scale (Bartley & Chute, 1969) was based on the clinician's rating of the patient's physical appearance, including such items as "unsteady voice," "sullen (or listless) face," and "spiritless eyes." However, patients with fatiguing illnesses, including CFS, often do not show external signs of fatigue and may appear superficially healthy or normal. To date, no reliable behavioral or physical signs of abnormal fatigue have been established. In the absence of objective measures, the patient's perception of his or her fatigue has become the focus of fatigue measures. Fortunately, recently developed multicomponent measures of subjectively experienced fatigue, modeled after the measurement of other subjective states (e.g., pain, anxiety) have multiple applications in clinical and research settings.

TABLE 5.1

Fatigue Rating Scales

Scale	Description	Response format	No. of items	Strengths/Limitations
Fatigue intensity measure				
Piper Fatigue Scale (Piper, Lindsey, Dodd, Ferketich, & Paul, 1989)	Seven dimensions of fatigue, including 3 intensity dimensions	VAS	42	Multidimensional measure/Respondents' difficulty with VAS format; not validated in chronic fatigue patients
Fatigue Scale (Chalder, Berelowitz, Pawlikowska, Watts, & Wessely, 1993)	Measure of "mental" and "physical" fatigue	VRS	14	Treatment sensitivity/Does not differentiate CFS & primary depression
Energy/Fatigue Scale (J. E. Ware & Sherbourne, 1992)	Brief measure of energy and fatigue	VRS	5	Ease of administration/ Floor effects in severely fatigued patients
VAS-F (Lee, Hicks, & Nino-Murcia, 1991)	Measure of energy and fatigue	VAS	18	Convergent and discriminant validity/ Fatigue and sleepiness confounded
Rhoten Fatigue Scale (Rhoten, 1982)	Single energy/ fatigue item	NRS	1	Ease of administration/ Inadequate validation data
Fatigue/Function measure				
Fatigue Severity Scale (Krupp et al., 1989)	Measure of effect of activities on functioning	VRS	9	Good validation data/ Possible ceiling effects with severe fatigue
Fatigue Assessment Instrument (Schwartz, Jandorf, & Krupp, 1993)	Measure of effect of activities on functioning	VRS	29	Measures important behavioral aspects of fatigue/Limited research track record
Multidimensional Assessment of Fatigue (Belza, Henke, Yelin, Epstein, & Gillis, 1993)	Measure of 5 dimensions of fatigue, including impact on daily activities	VAS or VRS	16	Brief, yet thorough in scope/No data on construct validity
Fatigue Impact Scale (Fisk, Ritvo, Ross, Haase, & Marrie, 1994)	Measure of cognitive, physical, & social functioning in relation to fatigue	VRS	40	Differentiates CFS from MS/Considerable overlap with depression symptoms

Continued next page

| TABLE 5.1 *(Continued)* |

Fatigue Rating Scales

Scale	Description	Response format	No. of items	Strengths/Limitations
Fatigue/Function measure *(continued)*				
Multidimensional Fatigue Inventory (Smets, Garssen, Bonke, & de Haes, 1995)	Measure of 5 fatigue dimensions, including reduced activity	VRS	20	Diagnostic and construct validity/1 subscale dimension approximates anhedonia, not fatigue
Fatigue/Affect measure				
Profile of Fatigue-Related States (Ray, Weir, Phillips, & Cullen, 1992)	Measure of 4 fatigue dimensions, including emotional distress	VRS	54	Comprehensive measure of CFS subjective states/ Discriminant validity of dimensions may be questionable
Profile of Mood States (McNair, Lorr, & Droppleman, 1992)	Measure of 6 dimensions, including emotional, fatigue, and confusion states	VRS	65	Adequate convergent validity of fatigue and vigor subscales/Length and poor discriminant validity of dimensions

Note: VAS = Visual analog scale; VRS = verbal rating scale; NRS = numerical rating scale.

Although several scales are now available that measure perception and severity of fatigue, many of these instruments remain untested in patients with CFS. For all assessments domains, the type and extent of the evaluation is dependent on the clinical setting or research project. Many of the fatigue measures described herein have been recently developed for specific medical conditions and therefore do not have substantial track records as general application clinical instruments. This chapter critically reviews fatigue intensity scales, fatigue–function measures, and fatigue–affect assessments (see Table 5.1), and it concludes with recommendations about the use of fatigue scales for clinicians and researchers.

Fatigue Intensity Scales

There is no "gold standard" of fatigue intensity to confirm the adequacy of any particular scale. Rather, the construct of fatigue intensity is often validated against other fatigue measures or functional impairment measures. Selecting a fatigue intensity scale may become a matter of the practical issues of participant comprehension and ease of administration and scoring.

The following description of response formats in fatigue scales is adapted from Karoly and Jensen (1987, pp. 42–46). Measures of fatigue intensity or severity will have one of the following response formats: a verbal rating scale (VRS), a visual analog scale (VAS), or a numerical rating scale (NRS). A VRS is a list of adjectives that describes different levels of fatigue intensity, such as mild and moderate. The VRS is easy to administer and score, easy for the respondent to comprehend, and compliance is good (Karoly & Jensen, 1987).

The VAS consists of a straight line, usually 10 cm long, whose ends are defined as the extreme limits of fatigue. For example, one end may be defined as *no fatigue*, whereas the other may be defined as *fatigue as bad as it could be*. To quantify responses, patients are asked to make a mark across the 10-cm line at the point that best indicates perceived severity. To score, the distance from the nonfatigued end to the mark provided by the patient is measured. This distance defines the patient's fatigue intensity score.

The problems with the VAS include (a) the patient's potential difficulty estimating fatigue in terms of distance on a line, (b) the extra time required by the assessor to measure the VAS distance, and (c) older patients' greater difficulty using the VAS (Karoly & Jensen, 1987). Given these problems, we suggest using validated measures of fatigue severity with a VRS response format. In a fatigue test validation study (Belza, 1995), a change in response format from a VAS to a VRS did not weaken internal consistency.

The NRS is a third method of fatigue intensity evaluation that instructs the patients to provide a single rating of their fatigue on a 0-to-10 or a 0-to-100 scale. The 0 point indicates *no fatigue* and the 10 or 100 point indicates *fatigue as bad as it could be*. The number chosen by the patient signifies the fatigue intensity for the patient. NRSs of fatigue in CFS (Deale et al., 1997; Sharpe et al., 1996) have shown sensitivity to treatment effects. NRSs are easier to understand and use than VASs and are extremely easy to administer and score.

PIPER FATIGUE SCALE (PFS)

The PFS (Piper et al., 1989) is a 42-item visual analogue scale designed to evaluate seven dimensions of fatigue, including a temporal dimension (e.g., duration), an intensity/severity dimension, an affective dimension, and a sensory dimension. The PFS is the first modern fatigue scale to subdivide the experience of fatigue into several distinct dimensions. These dimensions may be useful in developing a more sophisticated conceptualization of this complex subjective state. The initial validation study of the PFS (Piper et al., 1989) was conducted on 50 cancer patients starting their first week of outpatient radiation therapy. Twenty-four percent of these patients reported difficulties in responding to the VAS format. Eight patients were dropped from the study because of unanswered questions on the PFS. Internal consistency for the entire measure was a strong .85.

Content validity was determined by a panel of 11 fatigue experts. Convergent validity was shown between the affective dimension of the PFS and the affective subscales of the Profile of Mood States (POMS). However, the fatigue/inertia subscale of the POMS was also moderately correlated with both the affective dimension and total score on the PFS. Thus, the discriminant validity of the PFS was not supported.

Furthermore, participants in the testing sample for the PFS reported that their fatigue was more likely to be mild, intermittent, and acute rather than continuous or chronic. Therefore, the applicability of the PFS to a chronic fatigue population could not be evaluated. Finally, the length of the PFS combined with some participants' difficulties in using a VAS suggests that the PFS is impractical for quick assessment in clinical and research settings.

FATIGUE SCALE (FS)

The FS is a 14-item fatigue intensity measure (Chalder et al., 1993) with a four-choice response format that was developed with a sample of 374 general medical outpatients. The scale showed strong internal consistency. Factor analysis of the FS yielded two dimensions, physical and mental fatigue. Physical fatigue referred to items such as "I get tired easily," "I can no longer start anything," and "I feel weak," whereas mental fatigue encompassed difficulties with concentration and memory. The FS has shown sensitivity to treatment changes (S. Butler et al., 1991; Deale et al., 1997). Optimal sensitivity and specificity of the FS were determined with ROC analysis using the fatigue item on the Clinical Interview Schedule as the "gold standard."

The limitations of the FS include its inability to distinguish between CFS and primary depression patients (Wessely & Powell, 1989), an important diagnostic issue in CFS. Also, the questions comprising mental fatigue subscale describe cognitive difficulties rather than mental fatigue, which may or may not be associated with cognitive difficulties (Ray, Weir, Phillips, & Cullen, 1992). As such, the mental fatigue subscale may be more appropriately used as a rapid assessment device for subjective cognitive complaints. Another brief mental fatigue questionnaire (Bentall, Wood, Marrinan, Deans, & Edwards, 1993) also contains cognitive difficulty items such as "spells of confusion" and "poor concentration." Although the nine-item test discriminated between CFS and normals, it also failed to differentiate CFS and depression groups.

ENERGY/FATIGUE SCALE (EF)

Another verbal rating scale of fatigue intensity, the EF scale (J. E. Ware & Sherbourne, 1992) consists of five questions with a five-choice response format containing adjectives describing both fatigue *(worn out, tired)* and energy *(pep, energy)*. The EF scale, derived from the Rand Vitality Index (J. E. Ware, Johnston, & Davies-Avery, 1979) , was given to 2,389 adults visiting ambulatory medical clinics. The measure showed good internal consistency. When scores on the EF scale were correlated with single questions reflecting other subjective states, including sleep, anxiety, and positive affect, the correlations ranged from .37 to .54, as compared with correlations ranging from .68 to .78 for items on the hypothesized EF scale. However, no data were presented to show their relation to depression measures, an issue of major importance in establishing discriminant validity.

Although the sensitivity of the EF scale to the impact of disease and the effects of treatment has been claimed for clinical trials (Ware & Sherbourne, 1992) involving patients with hypertension (Croog et al., 1986), prostate disease (Fowler, Wennberg, & Timothy, 1988), and AIDS (Wachtel, Piette, & Mor, 1992; Wu et al., 1991), an examination of these studies revealed that two of them (Fowler et al., 1988; Wachtel et al., 1992) did not use the EF scale. The hypertension study (Croog et al., 1986) did not statistically separate the EF scale from a larger questionnaire, thus precluding assessments for treatment sensitivity or disease effects specific to this fatigue measure. In the remaining study cited in support of the EF scale (Wu et al., 1991), discriminant validity was demonstrated. That is, the EF scale showed lower correlations with other health perception scales on the MOS-SF-36 (Medical Outcome Study Scale; J. E. Ware & Sherbourne, 1992) than the correlations representing internal consistency within the EF scale.

The brevity of the EF scale may lead to floor effects in severely disabling illnesses (McHorney, Ware, Wu, & Sherbourne, 1994) such as CFS. No published study has specifically tested the psychometric properties of the EF scale in CFS.

VAS-F

A VAS of fatigue intensity, the VAS-F (Lee, Hicks, & Nino-Murcia, 1991) was initially tested on 57 patients presenting to a sleep disorders clinic for evaluation and on 75 healthy controls. The 18 items were selected from adjectives used in the literature and by people complaining of fatigue. Initially, the healthy participants rated their fatigue on the 18-item list before and after one night's sleep. Thirteen items describe fatigue states and five items list energy states. The internal consistency was excellent within each subscale of the VAS-F. Furthermore, both subscales were moderately to strongly correlated with the fatigue and vigor scales of the POMS, but not significantly correlated with the POMS scales of depression, tension, or anger. Thus, the VAS-F showed convergent as well as discriminant validity. The VAS-F was also strongly correlated with the Stanford Sleepiness Scale.

However, the VAS has been criticized (Chambers & Docktor, 1993) for using sleep disorder patients for whom perceptions of sleepiness and fatigue may be confounded. Given the importance of sleep disturbances as a differential diagnosis for CFS, the distinction between the constructs of sleepiness and fatigue is a significant concern (Chambers & Docktor, 1993; Krupp et al., 1991). Furthermore, evening fatigue scores for the patients were significantly lower than those of control participants, whereas morning fatigue scores were not significantly different between the groups. Thus, the essential diagnostic validity of the VAS was not demonstrated (Chambers & Docktor, 1993).

RHOTEN FATIGUE SCALE (RFS)

Finally, the RFS (Rhoten, 1982) is a 10-point NRS, with 0 equaling *total exhaustion* and 10 representing *not tired, peppy.* This scale was developed for use with postsurgical patients. The reliability data for the RFS were very limited, and patients were not tested against healthy controls. A reported correlation between investigators' ranking of fatigue and patient ratings was not specified.

Fatigue/Function Measures

Fatigue/function scales quantify the linkage between perceived fatigue intensity and functional limitations. Measuring the effect of fatigue on function is considered by some researchers (Canadian Research Group, 1987) to be more informative about specific fatigue-related dysfunction than is a fatigue intensity measure or a generic functional status measure. For instance, fatigue-related disabilities have been shown in one study (Fisk, Ritvo, Ross, Haase, & Marrie, 1994) to be a significantly greater perceived cause of incapacity in CFS than in MS, although no differences were found in overall functioning between the two groups on a generic functional status instrument.

Clearly, two patients with similar levels of fatigue severity in CFS may show widely divergent levels of incapacity. Conversely, two patients with similar functional limitations may show substantially different levels of fatigue severity. The following fatigue/function measures attempt to specify the important relationship between the symptom of fatigue and function level.

FATIGUE SEVERITY SCALE (FSS)

The FSS (Krupp et al., 1989) is composed of nine items with a seven-point response format. The items were initially selected on the basis of their ability to identify common features of fatigue in both MS and systemic lupus erythematosis (SLE). In the initial validation study (Krupp et al., 1989), patients with MS and SLE were compared with healthy adults. Internal consistency for the FSS was high for both illness groups. The scale clearly distinguished patients from controls, and it was moderately correlated ($r = .68$) with a single-item VAS of fatigue intensity. Also, treatment sensitivity was shown in a small sample of patients with Lyme disease before and after antibiotic therapy and in two MS patients treated with pemoline, a central nervous system stimulant. In all patients, clinical improvement in fatigue was associated with reductions in FSS scores. Mild to moderate correlations (.20–.46) were reported between the FSS and Center for Epidemiologic Studies–Depression Scale (CES-D) depression scores in MS, SLE, and control groups.

In subsequent studies of CFS patients (Friedberg & Krupp, 1994; Pepper et al., 1993) FSS scores were significantly higher in CFS than in MS and depression (Pepper et al., 1993), and FSS scores were sensitive to therapeutic change in CFS patients with high levels of comorbid depressive symptomatology (Friedberg & Krupp, 1994). In addition to its adequate psychometric properties, the FSS is a practical measure because of its brevity and ease of administration and scoring. On the other hand, a ceiling effect in the FSS (Friedberg & Krupp, 1994; Pepper et al., 1993) may limit its utility to assess severe fatigue-related disability, and therefore, the true association between the FSS and other health-related measures may be underestimated.

The Fatigue Assessment Instrument (FAI; Schwartz, Jandorf, & Krupp, 1993) is an expanded 29-item version of the FSS that assesses fatigue severity, situation specificity, the psychological consequences of fatigue, and whether fatigue responds to rest or sleep. Because of the length of the FAI, as well as the limited validation data, the FSS would be the preferred instrument for clinical and research applications.

MULTIDIMENSIONAL ASSESSMENT OF FATIGUE (MAF)

The MAF scale (Belza, 1995; Belza, Henke, Yelin, Epstein, & Gillis, 1993; Tack, 1990a, 1990b) contains 16 items and measures five dimensions of fatigue: degree, severity, the effects of stress, impact on activities of daily living, and timing. In two MAF validation studies using middle-aged and elderly patients with rheumatoid arthritis (Belza,1995; Belza et al., 1993), the internal consistency on the MAF was high. Furthermore, the MAF showed strong concurrent validity with the POMS fatigue subscale ($r > .75$) and divergent validity with the vigor subscale ($r \geq -.60$).

A change in response format on the MAF (Belza, 1995) from a VAS to a 10-point NRS did not affect internal consistency and, according to the author, obviated the problem of unclear markings. MAF scores were moderately correlated with scores on the POMS depression scale ($r = .47$) and the overall functioning score ($r = .56$) on the Health Assessment Questionnaire.

Two of the MAF items have strong face validity because they reflect CFS specific limitations related to impairments in walking and other exercise. Also, the MAF covers a comprehensive range of impairments from bathing and dressing to work and exercise, thus minimizing ceiling effects for severely disabled respondents. Overall, the MAF is brief yet thorough in scope.

On the other hand, three MAF items may be difficult for respondents to distinguish: Item 1 asks "to what degree" the participant has experienced fatigue, whereas item 2 asks "how severe" was the individual's fatigue over the previous week. The final item asks "how often" the individual was fatigued over the previous week. Clearly, the last item refers to frequency of fatigue, but the item asking about "degree" of fatigue may be interpreted as frequency or intensity, which may be confused further with the second item asking for a fatigue severity rating. Respondent misinterpretation of these items may distort MAF scores. Finally, the construct validity of the five dimensions of the MAF has not been confirmed with factor analysis, an essential task in the development of any multicomponent measure.

FATIGUE IMPACT SCALE (FIS)

The FIS (Fisk et al., 1994) also examines patients' perceptions of their functional limitations attributed to fatigue. It contains 10 cognitive function items, 10 physical function items, and 20 psychosocial function items. Each item is rated on a five-point Likert scale, 0 = *no problem* and 4 = *extreme problem*. The study sample included patients with CFS ($n = 141$), mild hypertension ($n = 34$), and probable or definite MS ($n = 105$). Internal consistency was very high (Cronbach's $\alpha = .98$) for the entire test. Significant differences in FIS scores, both overall and subscale scores, were found between all three groups, with CFS patients scoring highest on the total and on all subscale scores. However, the scores on the Sickness Impact Profile did not significantly differ between MS and CFS groups, indicating that the dysfunction attributed to symptoms of fatigue was significantly greater in the CFS group.

The ability of the FIS to discriminate between CFS and MS—both severely fatiguing medical illnesses that have been confused diagnostically—is an important strength; however, its ability to distinguish symptoms of depression from CFS was not examined. This is an especially important issue in the FIS because the 20-item psychosocial dimension subscale contains numerous items that may reflect depression and anxiety, as well as CFS symptoms, for example: "Because of my fatigue, I am more moody"; "Because of my fatigue, I am less motivated to engage in social activities"; "Because of my fatigue, I avoid situations that are stressful for me." Also, the FIS is relatively long compared with the other fatigue/function measures.

MULTIDIMENSIONAL FATIGUE INVENTORY (MFI-20)

The MFI-20 (Smets, Garssen, Bonke, & de Haes, 1995; Smets, Garssen, Cull, & de Haes, 1996) is a 20-item self-report instrument organized in five scales: general fatigue, physical fatigue, reduced activity, reduced motivation, and mental fatigue. A five-point true–not true response dimension gauges to what extent the particular statement applies to the individual. The instrument was tested in cancer patients ($n = 11$), CFS patients ($n = 357$), psychology students ($n = 481$), medical students ($n = 158$), army recruits ($n = 316$), and junior physicians ($n = 46$; Smets et al., 1995). The hypothesized five dimensions of the MFI were supported with a confirmatory factor analysis, and internal consistency within each dimension was adequate. Significant differences between groups were found for all subscales. Chronic fatigue patients showed the highest scores on all dimensions.

The limitations of the MFI-20 are as follows: The reduced motivation subscale approximates an anhedonia dimension and thus may be more closely associated with depression than with CFS. This possibility was not addressed in the MFI validation study. Second, the four-item mental fatigue subscale includes both cognitive difficulty and mental effort items that may be distinct constructs (Ray, Weir, Phillips, & Cullen, 1992). The sensitivity of the MFI to treatment changes has not been reported.

Is Fatigue Qualitatively Different in CFS?

The above fatigue/function scales have confirmed that subjectively rated fatigue severity is higher in CFS than in other fatiguing illnesses. However, severity measures do not address qualitative aspects of the fatigue experience. CFS patients often describe unusual fatigue sensations that, according to a recent descriptive study of 313 CFS patients (Dechene et al., 1994), may be useful in diagnosing the illness. A 19-item self-report Qualitative Fatigue Scale (QFS) contains descriptions of fatigue symptoms commonly found in a variety of medical conditions that may be associated with CFS, including subclinical hypothyroidism, glycogen storage disease, and mitochondrial dysfunction. Sample items include "My arms feel 'heavy' and 'dead' when I'm not moving them," "Climbing stairs feels like swimming against a strong current of molasses," and "I have to consciously think about a movement and concentrate before I can complete it."

A discriminant analysis using QFS scores correctly classified 91–97% of self-identified CFS patients and healthy significant others. By contrast, a self-report inventory of CFS symptoms based on the U.S. case definition (Fukuda et al., 1994) correctly classified only 67% of these patients and 85% of healthy significant others. Furthermore, the QFS was only weakly correlated with the CES-D, indicating the absence of a confound between these unusual fatigue symptoms and depression symptoms. A replication of these findings would be necessary to confirm the potential utility of the QFS in diagnostic evaluations of CFS.

Fatigue/Affect Assessments

Two multidimensional measures of fatigue and emotional states, the Profile of Fatigue-Related Symptoms (PFRS; Ray, Weir, Phillips, & Cullen, 1992) and the POMS (McNair, Lorr, & Droppleman, 1992) were developed to assess fatigue symptoms and negative emotional states in patients with CFS and psychiatric disorder, respectively.

PROFILE OF FATIGUE-RELATED SYMPTOMS (PFRS)

The PFRS (Ray, Weir, Phillips, & Cullen, 1992) was developed from a 96-item symptom questionnaire given to two samples of CFS patients (n_1 = 208 and n_2 = 147). Items in the initial questionnaire listed symptoms that have been commonly described in the literature on CFS. A principal components analysis yielded four factors accounting for 48.3% of the variance in Study 1 and 51.2% in Study 2. The final scales included a total of 54 items. The four scales were labeled Emotional Distress, Cognitive Difficulty, Fatigue, and Somatic Symptoms. Convergent validity was demonstrated between the fatigue scale of the PFRS and the fatigue severity scale (r = .65; Krupp et al., 1989). The internal consistency of each of the four scales was high, and test–retest reliability over several hours in a separate group of 48 patients yielded very high correlations (.86–.95). The authors noted that CFS symptoms may fluctuate substantially from day to day, and therefore, a longer test–retest interval may have been inappropriate.

Although the four scales of the PFRS were factorially distinct, moderate correlations (.44–.64) were found between the scales; this finding does not support the discriminant validity of these dimensions. The authors pointed out that the significant interrelationships of symptom dimensions may reflect an underlying dimension of physical and psychological stress (Watson & Pennebaker, 1989) that may exert an important, if not primary, influence on symptom experience.

Because the PFRS was constructed from the responses of CFS patients, it is more likely to provide an accurate representation of the CFS symptom experience. This multidimensional instrument can be recommended as an adequately validated measure of CFS symptoms, although CFS researchers tend to use their own (unvalidated) questionnaires to assess CFS symptoms. If future use of the PFRS confirms its efficiency in capturing the symptom experience of CFS, then it may become a preferred alternative to unvalidated measures.

PROFILE OF MOOD STATES (POMS)

The POMS (McNair et al., 1992) is a 65-item multidimensional self-report measure composed of six subscales: tension–anxiety (T), depression–dejection (D), anger–hostility (A), vigor–activity (V), fatigue–inertia (F), and confusion–bewilderment (C). Reliability and validity studies have been reported (McNair et al., 1992). The POMS fatigue–inertia subscale was strongly correlated with the fatigue subscale of the PFRS and moderately correlated with the FSS ($r = .59$; Ray, Weir, Phillips, & Cullen, 1992). Thus, the fatigue subscale showed adequate convergent validity with other fatigue measures.

The POMS has been used in three CFS studies: a cross-sectional psychiatric assessment (Millon, Fernando, Blaney, Morgan, & Mantero-Atienza, 1989) and two unsuccessful controlled treatment trials (Lloyd et al., 1993; Straus, Dale, Tobi, et al., 1988). The measure has been shown to be sensitive to psychosocial intervention in cancer patients (Fawzy, Cousins, Fawzy, & Kemeny, 1990). However, in multi-instrument assessment protocols, the length of the POMS (65 items) may limit its use with physically ill populations. A shorter 37-item version of the POMS (POMS-SF), developed by Curran, Andrykowski, and Studts (1983) has shown comparable internal consistency to the original POMS. Furthermore, correlations between total mood disturbance and subscales scores on the POMS-SF and those from the original POMS all exceeded .95. The POMS-SF may be considered an alternative to the original POMS when a brief measure of psychological distress is desired with a subscale assessment for fatigue.

Although the POMS has a 15-year track record of use in a variety of normal and clinical populations, it is not yet clear that a 65-item measure is necessary to assess dimensions that are not independent and that may in fact represent a general factor of emotional distress. Correlations between scales of the POMS are as high as .77 (McNair et al., 1992), although the fatigue–inertia dimension was only moderately correlated ($r = .41$) with the three affective dimensions.

Fatigue Scale Recommendations

Psychometric considerations suggest the use of fatigue scales that (a) have been diagnostically validated in CFS and depression samples, (b) assess several factorially distinct dimensions of fatigue, and (c) are easy to administer and score. Unfortunately, none of the measures discussed meet all of these criteria. Instead, we will make recommendations based on our own clinical and research experience with fatigue measures. For the clinician, the FSS or the MAF provides a rapid assessment of fatigue-related impairments. For the researcher, the selection of any two fatigue instruments may offer (a) a more thorough description of the fatigue experience and (b) an opportunity for concurrent validation of each scale, as well as convergent and discriminant validation with other measures.

Psychometric Evaluation | 6

n 1992, the National Institute of Mental Health and the National Institute of Allergy and Infectious Diseases sponsored a conference on guidelines for CFS research (Schluederberg et al., 1992) that recommended the evaluation of six behavioral and psychosocial domains: fatigue, mood disturbance, functional status, sleep disturbance, global well-being (i.e., psychiatric status), and pain. Behavioral coping and social support may also be important in a comprehensive CFS evaluation. Although the conference offered suggestions for the use of specific instruments for some of these domains, little information has been available to guide the choice of measures. This chapter will examine and critique psychometric instruments used in the assessment of CFS, including measures of depression, functional level, global psychiatric status, coping, social support, health locus of control, subjective pain, somatic perception, and illness behavior and attribution. The CFS researcher may find this review helpful in guiding the choice of instruments for psychometric evaluations and clinical or naturalistic outcome research. This chapter also assists clinicians in choosing one or two selected measures to complement initial and outcome assessments for their CFS patients. Significantly, these measures may reveal clinical issues that are not evident from therapy sessions alone.

The majority of psychometric instruments used in the assessment of CFS have not been validated in CFS samples, and therefore it cannot be certain that their content and structure are fully appropriate to this illness (Ray, Weir,

Phillips, & Cullen, 1992). Furthermore, the most comprehensive instruments are lengthy, and their completion may be particularly onerous for a group of patients who fatigue easily.

Another problem with psychometric evaluation in CFS is that the measures cannot distinguish whether identified psychopathology is a cause, effect, or covariate of CFS symptomatology. Thus, conclusions about etiology that are based on self-report measures should be viewed with skepticism. However, psychometric assessment may be valuable in quantifying differences in clinical presentations. For example, patients who meet symptom criteria for CFS may range in disability from those who appear indistinguishable from healthy adults to other patients who suffer bed-bound disability.

Depression Rating Scales

In psychodiagnostic studies, CFS is most commonly associated with depression diagnoses or elevated depressive symptomatology (Friedberg, 1996a). Therefore, the assessment and differential diagnosis of depression in CFS is a crucial issue. Overlap symptoms between the two disorders, including fatigue, sleep disturbance, and concentration difficulty, require careful consideration when using a standardized measure of depression. It is possible that endorsement of these symptoms on a depression scale may result in the overestimation of depressive symptomatology in CFS patients. Furthermore, the sole use of self-report measures to establish depression diagnoses precludes clinical judgment of endorsed symptoms as depression related or CFS related.

Several brief depression rating scales, including the Beck Depression Inventory (BDI), the CES-D, the Zung Self-Rating Depression Scale (SDS), and the Hamilton Rating Scale for Depression have long track records in the assessment of depressive symptomatology in psychiatric and medical patients. However, none of these scales has been standardized for use in fatiguing illnesses. Thus, the validity of these measures must often be extrapolated from the community-based testing samples and psychiatric patients used in developing these scales.

The 21-item BDI (Beck, 1967) may overestimate depression in CFS because of the significant number of items related to somatic functioning. In a comparative study of CFS, MS, and depression (S.K. Johnson et al., 1996b), 53% of nondepressed CFS patients scored above the depression cut score (10) on the BDI. This spurious elevation of scores reflected endorsement of a higher percentage of somatic items. In another study using the BDI as a screening instrument for depression in CFS (Farmer et al., 1996), the use of higher threshold scores (14 and 20) for depression diagnoses did not alleviate the problem of misdiagnosis. The rate of depression misclassification in this study ranged from 36 to 38% in a sample of 95 CFS patients (Farmer et al., 1996). Because of the high risk of false-positive cases, the clinical diagnosis of depression on the BDI should not be based solely on a cutoff score.

The CES-D (Radloff, 1977), a 20-item depression rating scale, also contains several items that overlap with CFS, although several studies of the CES-D in medical populations suggest that the biasing effect of the somatic items is modest (e.g., Blalock, DeVellis, Brown, & Wallston, 1989). For certain illness groups such as chronic pain (Turk & Okifuji, 1994), a higher cutoff score for depression may restore its validity as a screening instrument for depression. However, in a well-designed investigation of the diagnostic efficiency of the CES-D in 425 primary medical outpatients (Fechner-Bates, Coyne, & Schwenk, 1994), the positive predictive value (i.e., the probability that a patient obtaining a positive screening score [CES-D ≥ 16] will have a depression diagnosis) was a modest 27.9%. Also, one fifth of the participants with scores below 16 met criteria for major depressive disorder. Given the inconsistent findings for the CES-D in evaluating depression in medical illness, we do not recommend it for CFS patients.

Both the Zung SDS (Zung, 1965) and the clinician-administered Hamilton Rating Scale for Depression (Hamilton, 1967) measure the presence and severity of depressive symptoms. On both scales, 30–40% of the items are reflective of CFS symptomatology, and therefore it is more likely that depression scores will be artificially inflated. The validity of these scales as depression screening instruments in CFS has not been evaluated.

A rating scale developed for medical patients, the Hospital Anxiety and Depression Scale (HADS; Zigmond & Snaith, 1983), consists of two 8-item subscales: one relating to depression and the other to anxiety. The authors intentionally excluded from the scale all items that might relate either to somatization of mood or to physical illness, such as headaches, dizziness, and loss of appetite. Evidence was provided to show that the subscale scores of the HADS were relatively little affected by physical illness and moderately correlated with interview-based assessments. However, the internal consistency of the two subscales of the HADS was poor. Also, one item—"I feel as if I am slowed down"—is contained on the depression scale, which may arguably be endorsed by CFS patients as a symptom of their fatigue rather than depression.

The HADS has been used in several psychological studies of CFS (e.g., Ray et al., 1995b) and has shown sensitivity to treatment effects in CFS (Sharpe et al., 1996). However, in a recent clinical study of medical patients (Silverstone, 1994), the positive predictive value of the HADS for a diagnosis of major depressive disorder was only 17%, whereas in a study of geriatric medical inpatient sample (Davies, Burn, McKenzie, & Brothwell, 1993), the HADS proved unsuitable as a case finding or screening instrument because of a high incidence of missed cases. It appears that the HADS, in contrast to the aforementioned depression rating scales, underestimates the true prevalence of depression in medical patient populations.

The research literature on the assessment of depression in medical illness has indicated that somatic symptoms, including fatigue, are not sensitive to the diagnosis of depression in medical populations (Abbey, Toner, Garfinkel, Kennedy, & Kaplan, 1990; Frank et al., 1992; Plumb & Holland, 1977). Rather, cognitive–affective symptoms such as self-hate, suicidal ideation, and indecisiveness have been found to be the best discriminators of depression in medical conditions such as cancer (Plumb & Holland, 1977); spinal cord injury and rheumatoid arthritis (Frank et al., 1992); and end-stage renal disease, irritable bowel syndrome, postinfectious neuromyalgia, and eating disorders (Abbey et al., 1990).

In contrast, a comparative study of CFS, MS, and primary depression (S.K. Johnson et al., 1996b) revealed that the best indicator of major depressive disorder in CFS patients was higher scores on the mood category items of the BDI. (Depression diagnoses were based on the Diagnostic Inteview Schedule [DIS].) Furthermore, CFS was best differentiated from primary depression patients by BDI items labeled "self-reproach" symptoms (lower in CFS) and somatic symptoms (higher in CFS). Perhaps the BDI could be recommended for both clinical and research applications because it is the only depression rating scale to be empirically tested and interpreted for both depressed and nondepressed patients with CFS. Rather than relying on a single cutoff score for the BDI, scoring the mood, self-reproach, and somatic items separately (Huber, Freidenberg, Paulson, Shuttleworth, & Christy, 1990) may assist in differential diagnosis of depression in CFS. Ideally, a study comparing several depression rating scales in depressed and nondepressed CFS patients would yield a more definitive recommendation for the measure with the highest positive predictive value. In the absence of such information, the use of a clinician-administered psychiatric interview that allows for professional judgment in classifying overlap symptoms such as fatigue, sleep disturbance, and concentration difficulty is essential to confirm a diagnosis of depression in CFS.

Measures of Functional Status

KARNOFSKY PERFORMANCE SCALE (KPS)

The KPS (Karnofsky, Abelmann, Craver, & Burchenal, 1948) is a widely used 10-point functional status rating (0 = *dead* to 100 = *normal*) that emphasizes physical performance and dependency. Patients are assigned to categories on the KPS by a clinician. It is assumed that a patient with a low score because of immobility has a poorer quality of life than the patient with a higher score, and vice versa. The social, emotional, and symptom-related aspects of functioning are not included. Apart from its limited content, the clinician rating of patient functioning on the KPS may differ substantially from the patient's self-rating (Bowling, 1991).

The KPS has shown good interrater reliability (Mor, Lalibert, Morris, & Wienmann, 1984) as well as sensitivity to treatment change in a cognitive–behavioral treatment study of CFS patients (Sharpe et al., 1996). However, the scale's numeric status has not been seriously challenged, and it has generally been uncritically accepted and applied in a large number of clinical settings (Bowling, 1991). If used, the KPS should be augmented with other quality of life measures that sample a variety of physical activities and social behaviors.

SICKNESS IMPACT PROFILE (SIP)

The 136-item SIP (Deyo, Inui, Leininger, & Overman, 1982; Deyo & Inui, 1983) was developed as a measure of perceived health status for use as an outcome instrument in health care evaluation across a wide range of health problems and diseases. The SIP concentrates on assessing the impact of sickness on daily activities, behavior, feelings of emotional well-being, and social functioning. The 12 areas assessed are work, recreation, emotion, affect, home life, sleep, rest, eating, ambulation, mobility, communication, and social interaction. Both test–retest reliability and internal consistency are high on the SIP, and convergent and discriminant validity as well as sensitivity to treatment change have been demonstrated (Bowling, 1991). However, its construct validity as judged by factor analysis has not been studied. It may be self- or interviewer-administered and takes 20 to 30 minutes to complete. A practical limitation of the SIP is its length, given the impaired attention and mental fatigue often found in CFS patients.

MEDICAL OUTCOME STUDY SCALES (MOS)

The 60-item MOS scale, a broadly based measure of functional status, identifies six dimensions, including physical activities, mental health, social functioning, bodily pain, energy and fatigue, and perceptions of health (Brook et al., 1979). The measure records limitations caused by ill health on a scale of 0 (*limited in all activities, including basic self-care*) to 100 (*no limitations, able to carry out vigorous activities like running or strenuous sports*). A shortened 20-item version of the MOS (MOS-SF-20) has been developed (Stewart, Hays, & Ware, 1988), although a subsequent 36-item version (MOS-SF-36; J. E. Ware & Sherbourne, 1992) is more often used. Reliability and validity studies for the 20-item (Stewart et al., 1988) and the 36-item (McHorney, Ware, & Raczek, 1993; McHorney, Ware, Wu, & Sherbourne, 1994) versions of the MOS have shown adequate internal consistency, discriminant validity among subscales, and substantial differences between patient and nonpatient populations in the pattern of scores. The SF-36 has shown adequate psychometric properties as a measure of functional status in a CFS population (D. Buchwald, Pearlman, Umali, Schmaling, & Katon, 1996), and it has distinguished CFS from other fatiguing illnesses (D. Buchwald et al., 1996). A recent behavioral treatment study of CFS patients demonstrated that the SF-36 is sensitive to treatment change (Deale, Chalder, Marks, & Wessely, 1997).

A possible limitation of the MOS scales is relevant to CFS. In moderate to severely disabled patients, there may be a floor effect (indicating severe disability)—especially on the physical disability scales—because there are few items that distinguish among very low levels of functioning. For instance, there is only one item on daily self-care activities. The floor effect in very disabled patients will result in a loss of information about patient functioning and reduce the true variability of scores. In the SF-36 validation studies, cited above, floor effects were most likely to occur (61%) in patients with both psychiatric and medical conditions, paralleling the diagnostic complexities of CFS. In such cases, a measure that is more sensitive to physical disability, such as the KPS or the SIP, is recommended.

Global Measures of Psychiatric Status (or Well-Being)

Multidimensional measures of psychiatric symptomatology are designed to detect the presence of psychiatric disorder by using cutoff scores. Compared with structured diagnostic interviews, broadly based self-report measures of psychiatric status are generally less valid indicators of psychopathology (e.g., Morrison, Edwards, & Weissman, 1994). As in the measurement of depression, symptom overlap between psychiatric disorder and CFS may tend to inflate estimates of psychiatric co-morbidity determined by cutoff scores. This section reviews several such global measures, including the General Health Questionnaire, the MMPI, the SCL-90-R, the BSI, and the Millon clinical inventories.

GENERAL HEALTH QUESTIONNAIRE (GHQ)

The GHQ is a self-administered screening questionnaire designed for use in clinical settings in order to detect diagnosable psychiatric disorder (Goldberg, 1972). The four scales of the GHQ are somatic symptoms, anxiety and insomnia, social dysfunction, and severe depression. The GHQ is available in four versions ranging from 12 to 60 items. The more than 50 validation studies conducted on the GHQ have shown moderate to high levels of internal consistency and moderate correlations with psychiatric diagnoses (Bowling, 1991). It has been observed that physically ill people tend to score higher on the GHQ (Bridges & Goldberg, 1986; Finlay-Jones & Murphy, 1979), creating a problem of false positives when classifying people as psychiatric cases using a threshold score. In patients with chronic or acute medical illness, a cutting score of 11 (compared with the standard cutoff of 5) has been found to correlate best with psychiatric "caseness" (Bridges & Goldberg, 1986).

The 28-item version of the GHQ is more often used in studies of CFS (e.g., Blakely et al., 1991), although the GHQ 28 contains at least five symptoms that could be considered a direct result of the physical and cognitive impairments associated with CFS. A recent study of the GHQ in CFS patients (D. Buchwald, Pearlman, Kith, Katon, & Schmaling, 1997) found that a threshold score of 12 yielded the best sensitivity and specificity for current psychiatric diagnoses. However, a study of the GHQ as a screening instrument for psychiatric caseness in 95 individuals with CFS (Farmer et al., 1996) found that the GHQ performed poorly as a screener for psychiatric morbidity when compared with a structured psychiatric interview. Also, a substantial retest effect has been reported for the GHQ (Ormel, Koeter, & van den Brink, 1989): GHQ-reported symptom improvement for psychiatric outpatients contrasted with no reported change or deterioration on a structured clinical interview 5 months after initial assessment. The retest effect may reduce its usefulness in longitudinal population and outcome studies. In the absence of reference tables for retest effects, the GHQ should not be used as the sole psychiatric measure in prospective studies.

MINNESOTA MULTIPHASIC PERSONALITY INVENTORY (MMPI AND MMPI–2)

The MMPI, a widely used 566-item questionnaire with a true–false response format, is designed to assess the severity of several specific psychiatric conditions (Halfaway & McKinley, 1940, 1989). The test contains 10 clinical scales and three validity scales. In an investigation of the MMPI and MMPI-2 as predictors of psychiatric diagnosis in an outpatient sample (Morrison et al., 1994), a discriminant function analysis correctly classified only 49% and 50% of the cases for the MMPI and MMPI-2, respectively. These results suggested that MMPI findings alone should not be used as a basis for diagnostic decisions.

Despite many research attempts to distinguish functional and organic illness using the MMPI, no successful classification strategy has been established (Fiedler, Kipen, DeLuca, Kelly, & Natelson, 1996; Willcockson, 1985). Most commonly, clinically significant elevations on Scale 1 (Hypochondriasis) and Scale 3 (Hysteria) have been found in CFS patients (Blakely et al., 1991; Fiedler et al., 1996; Schmaling & Jones, 1996). These scales contain physical symptoms, including a number of CFS symptoms. Similarly, patients with chronic pain, MS, closed head injuries, and a mixed neurologic population also present clinical elevations on Scales 1 and 3 (Fiedler et al., 1996). In a comparative study of neurologic, psychiatric, and chronic pain patients using the MMPI (Cripe, Maxwell, & Hill, 1995), clinical inspection and discriminant function analyses of the clinical and research scales could not classify groups correctly, but discriminant function analyses of 37 neurologic symptom items correctly classified the groups with 78% overall accuracy. This study suggests that without complex statistical analyses, the MMPI is not a useful instrument to differentiate psychiatric and general medical conditions. Unfortunately, the popularity of the MMPI as a comprehensive clinical assessment instrument is often not tempered by its well-established limitations in medical populations.

Finally, the MMPI requires 1 to 3 hours of administration time, a significant consideration with impaired patients who have low energy. Rather than using the MMPI to generate psychiatric diagnoses, a brief structured psychiatric interview for depressive and anxiety disorders (e.g., the Schedule for Affective Disorders and Schizophrenia) may be a preferred alternative for the CFS patient. Such an interview will be less taxing for the patient and will yield more definitive diagnostic data.

SYMPTOM CHECKLIST–90–REVISED (SCL-90-R) AND BRIEF SYMPTOM INVENTORY (BSI)

The SCL-90-R (Derogatis, 1983) and a shorter 53-item subset of the 90 items, the BSI (Derogatis, 1975) are broadly based measures of psychological distress that yield three scores, the most sensitive being the Global Severity Index. Both the SCL-90-R and the BSI contain nine symptom dimensions: somatization, obsessive–compulsive, interpersonal sensitivity, depression, anxiety, hostility, phobic anxiety, paranoid ideation, and psychoticism. Both measures have high levels of internal consistency and show construct validity based on factor analysis of the nine hypothesized symptom constructs. However, the number of factor analytic symptom dimensions varies from one study to another, and intercorrelations range from about .40 to .90 (e.g., Rief & Fichter, 1992). It has been suggested (e.g., Bonynge, 1993) that the SCL-90-R more accurately reflects a single factorial dimension of generalized distress or discomfort rather than qualitatively distinct dimensions related to specific psychiatric disorders.

Both the SCL-90-R and the BSI are sensitive to treatment changes and are often used in treatment trials. However, 15–20% of the items describe physical and cognitive symptoms that overlap with CFS symptoms. In clinical outcome studies, comparisons can be made between subscales that are heavily weighted with CFS symptoms (e.g., somatization and obsessive–compulsive) and the remaining subscales in order to assess changes in psychiatric symptomatology versus changes in CFS phenomena. This strategy has been useful in the assessment of low-back pain patients (Bernstein, Jaremko, & Hinkley, 1994). In a comparison of cognitive–behavioral treatment for CFS and primary depression (Friedberg & Krupp, 1994), the BSI showed significant score reductions in the subgroup of treated CFS patients with higher levels of depressive symptomatology.

MILLON INVENTORIES

The Millon Clinical Multiaxial Inventory (MCMI, MCMI-II, and MCMI-III; T. Millon, 1987; Millon, Millon, & Davis, 1994) is a 175-item self-report questionnaire designed to assess Axis II personality disorders as well as Axis I pathology (McCann, 1990). The MCMI has been used in psychiatric studies of CFS (e.g., Pepper et al., 1993) to determine the presence of personality disorder diagnoses. Unfortunately, the MCMI-II has shown a high rate of false positives in a psychiatric outpatient population when compared with the Structured Clinical Interview for *DSM-III-R*, Axis II (Guthrie & Mobley, 1994). On the other hand, a negative test result in this study was usually an accurate indication that the participant did not have a personality disorder. The authors suggested that the MCMI-II should be considered a screening instrument for Axis II disorder, with positive results indicating the need for a more extensive evaluation.

Coping Measures

Coping is the process of executing a response to a perceived threat to oneself (Carver, Scheier, & Weintraub, 1989). The ongoing stress of an illness, such as CFS, triggers coping responses that may profoundly affect adaptation to diminished abilities and intrusive symptoms. Several psychological studies of CFS have incorporated coping measures, including the Ways of Coping scale (Blakeley et al., 1991; Lewis et al., 1994), the COPE (Coping Orientations to Problems Experienced; Antoni et al., 1994; Ray, Weir, Stewart, Miller, & Hyde, 1993) and the Illness Management Questionnaire (IMQ; Ray, Jefferies, & Weir, 1995a; Ray, Weir, Stewart, et al., 1993).

The Ways of Coping scale (WOC; Folkman & Lazarus, 1980), an empirically derived measure, distinguishes two general types of coping: (a) problem-focused coping, which is directed to problem solving or actively changing the source of stress, and (b) emotion-focused coping, which seeks to lessen or manage stress associated with a situation. Although most stressors elicit both types of coping, problem-focused coping tends to predominate when people feel that something constructive can be done, whereas emotion-focused coping tends to predominate when people feel the stressor must be endured. In a comparative study of CFS and irritable bowel syndrome (Lewis et al., 1994), the WOC revealed that CFS sufferers used significantly more confrontive coping, planful problem solving, and social support seeking rather than potentially stress-reducing emotion-focused strategies such as relaxation.

The COPE (Carver, Scheier, & Weintraub, 1989), a theoretically based coping inventory, is comprised of five conceptually distinct scales of problem-focused coping and five scales of emotion-focused coping, as well as three additional scales (e.g., venting of emotions). The authors of the COPE stated that a theory-based approach allows inclusion of scales to measure interesting aspects of coping that are less obviously related to the self-regulatory functions assessed by empirically derived coping measures. Two emotion-focused strategies measured by the COPE, denial and mental disengagement, have been associated with greater disturbances in both physical and psychosocial domains in CFS patients (Antoni et al., 1994).

In contrast to the WOC and the COPE, both of which included healthy individuals in their test construction sample, the Illness Management Questionnaire (IMQ; Ray, Weir, Stewart, et al., 1993) was empirically derived and validated with a sample of CFS patients. The IMQ yielded four factors: maintaining activity, accommodating the illness, focusing on symptoms, and information seeking. The IMQ was intended to provide a measure of coping that is problem focused rather than directed toward the management of distress. The scales containing behavioral strategies directly relevant to CFS were better predictors of impairment and emotional adjustment when compared with the COPE problem-focused scales, which were designed for more general application (Ray et al., 1993). Significantly, the IMQ scales suggest that coping strategies in CFS cannot be easily classified as adaptive or maladaptive. Rather, each strategy will produce a benefit as well as extract a cost. For instance, maintaining activity protects everyday functioning but at the cost of increased anxiety. On the other hand, accommodating the illness safeguards emotional adjustment, but at the expense of functional impairment.

A recent comparative study of the WOC, the COPE, and the Coping Strategy Indicator (Clark, Bormann, Cropanzano, & James, 1995) confirmed adequate construct validity for all of these measures and showed significant associations with external criteria, including hassles and uplifts, physical symptoms, satisfaction with life, and positive and negative affectivity.

Might coping strategies be altered by cognitive–behavioral interventions for CFS patients? Unfortunately, no coping measures have been used in CFS treatment studies. The IMQ captures the dynamic qualities of coping characteristic of a chronic, fluctuating illness such as CFS, but it does not assess emotion-focused coping. On the other hand, the COPE and the WOC address a broad range of coping activities, including emotion-focused strategies, but these measures may be less sensitive to the changing adaptational requirements of patients with chronic illness. Thus, the choice of coping inventory is somewhat arbitrary. Each scale will yield valuable information, but none of these measures alone will yield a comprehensive overview of coping in the CFS patient.

Measures of Social Support

Social support has rarely been evaluated in psychological investigations of CFS. Yet satisfaction with social support has been positively associated with functional impairment in one study (Schmaling & DiClementi, 1995), but negatively related to symptomatic relapse (Lutgendorf, Antoni, et al., 1995) in another CFS study. Other data suggest that low perceived social support prior to the onset of CFS may increase vulnerability to the illness (Lewis et al., 1994).

A 14-item measure of social support was developed by Ray (1992) and administered to 207 patients with CFS. A principal components analysis of the items revealed two factors: one related to others' positive attitudes and behaviors, and the other related to negative items concerning expressed irritation, criticism, conflicts, and misunderstanding from others. Positive support had a significant inverse relationship with anxiety, whereas negative support was directly related to both anxiety and depression. Neither scale was associated with functional impairment. Scores on this social support scale were not significantly correlated with any psychological variable, including anxiety and depression, in a group of long-term CFS patients (Friedberg et al., 1994).

Another social support measure, the Perceived Social Support Inventory (Procideno & Heller, 1983), contains 20 items representing two subscales, family and friends. It examines emotional, instrumental, and problem-solving support as obtained from each of the groups represented by these two subscales. Validation studies have been reported (Procideno & Heller, 1983).

Because the literature on social support in chronic illness, especially chronic pain, has shown the importance of this dimension as a correlate of functional status and emotional well-being (Keefe, Dunsmore, & Burnet, 1992), the measurement of social support in CFS populations may have important implications for clinical assessment and treatment.

Multidimensional Health Locus of Control Scales (MHLC: Form C)

Form C of the MHLC was developed to measure the illness-specific locus of control beliefs of people with an existing health problem (Wallston, 1989). An internal locus of control reflects a person's perceived responsibility for illness outcomes; an others' locus of control indicates reliance on others to control the illness; and a chance locus of control reflects the belief that changes in illness are determined by fate, chance, or luck. These three factors of the original MHLC were replicated in a recent study of CFS patients (Ray et al., 1995a), and the scales had alpha reliabilities of .79, .65, and .85, respectively.

Health locus of control measures have shown predictive utility for illness outcomes. Internal locus of control has been significantly correlated with measures of psychological growth and mastery in cardiac rehabilitation (Younger, Marsh, & Grap, 1995) and with the use of more active behavioral coping strategies and successful rehabilitation in low-back pain patients (Harkapaa, Jarvikoski, Mellin, Hurri,

& Luoma, 1991). MS patients with a predominately internal locus of control had more knowledge of their disease, practiced more self-care, and had a more benign course of their illness than did those with an external locus of control (Wassem, 1991). Furthermore, an internal locus of control predicted long-term clinical improvement in psychophysiological disorders (McLean & Pietroni, 1990). In contrast, pain patients with a chance orientation toward locus of control were more likely to report depression, anxiety, and obsessive–compulsive symptoms; to have higher overall levels of psychological distress; and to report feeling helpless to deal effectively with their pain problems (Crisson & Keefe, 1988). Finally, a review of the effects of psychological treatment on cancer patients (Trijsburg, Van Knippenberg, & Rijpma, 1992) found that tailored counseling was effective with respect to improving an internal health locus of control.

It has been suggested that attributing CFS to a presumably uncontrollable physical cause may relieve the person of responsibility for the illness, promote helplessness, and discourage recovery-oriented behaviors (S. Butler et al., 1991; Powell et al., 1990). Two studies have examined this hypothesis but failed to find support for it. No differences in health locus of control were found between groups of primary care patients with or without chronic fatigue (Cope, Mann, Pelosi, & David, 1996). Both cohorts reported a relative sense of responsibility and control over health. In addition, illness attributions in a descriptive study of CFS patients (Ray et al., 1995a) were unrelated to locus of control beliefs or to scores on a coping measure. It was suggested by the authors of the study that believing in responsibility for one's health does not necessarily entail a belief that one can, in practice, control it. Furthermore, locus of control beliefs do not imply a specific behavioral orientation (Wallston, 1992). However, the concept of taking responsibility for those health-related beliefs and behaviors that *can* be controlled is consistent with effective cognitive–behavioral interventions for the psychological and physical symptoms of chronic illness. The findings of a recent 1-year prospective study of outcome predictors in CFS (Ray, Jefferies, & Weir, 1997) suggested that interventions that enhanced perceived control could benefit the course of the illness.

Assessment of Subjective Pain

Although assessment of pain in CFS has been recommended in a NIH-sponsored conference on the definition and evaluation of CFS

(Schluederberg et al., 1992), we found no formal assessment of pain in any published study of CFS. The case definition of CFS includes symptom criteria of muscle and joint pain, which have been reported by the majority of CFS patients in two large sample descriptive studies (Friedberg, 1995c; Komaroff et al., 1996). Also, a majority of CFS patients either meet symptom criteria for fibromyalgia (D. Buchwald, Pascualy, Bombardier, & Kith, 1994) or report having fibromyalgia (Friedberg et al., 1994), a rheumatologic condition characterized by diffuse generalized pain. Two popular pain evaluation inventories may provide useful data in a comprehensive evaluation of pain in CFS patients.

WEST HAVEN–YALE MULTIDIMENSIONAL PAIN INVENTORY (MPI)

The MPI (Kerns, Turk, & Rudy, 1985) consists of 52 items on 13 empirically derived scales designed to measure the subjective experience and personal impact of pain on a patient's life. The administration time is approximately 20–30 minutes. This instrument has been found to be both valid and reliable in pain assessment (Kerns et al., 1985).

Using cluster analysis of MPI responses in chronic pain patients, Turk and Rudy (1988, 1990) identified three subgroups of patients: (a) The *dysfunctional* group showed high pain severity scores, interference in their lives due to pain, and psychological distress and lower perceptions of control and engagement in daily activities; (b) the *interpersonally distressed* group viewed their family and significant others as not supportive; and (c) the *minimizers/adaptive copers* reported lower ratings of pain severity and pain interference in their lives as well as higher levels of activity and perceptions of life control. Despite differences in medical diagnoses, the similar responses to pain in each subgroup suggest that they may benefit from similar psychosocial interventions (Keefe et al., 1992). The concept of psychiatrically distinct subgroups may be applicable to CFS. A descriptive study of 565 CFS patients (Hickie et al., 1995) revealed two qualitatively distinct subsets of CFS patients: a high symptom severity/high disability subgroup and a low symptom severity/low disability subgroup. Scores on a psychiatric symptom measure and ratings of depression- and anxiety-related disability were significantly higher in the high symptom severity subgroup.

MCGILL PAIN QUESTIONNAIRE (MPQ)

The MPQ (Melzack, 1983) is a widely used pain instrument consisting of three major classes of word descriptors that are identified by patients to describe their pain. The four components of the test include (a) a human figure drawing on which patients are asked to mark the location of their pain; (b) a series of 78 adjectives divided into 20 groups from which patients identify their experience by circling word descriptors; (c) questions about prior pain experience, pain location, and information about the use of pain medication; and (d) a present pain intensity index. The MPQ is the first pain inventory to identify pain as a multidimensional construct, although it has been criticized in regard to its reliability, construct validity, and ability to discriminate between diagnostic groups (Tollison & Hinnant, 1996). It also requires patients to have a relatively high level of reading ability and intelligence. The administration time is approximately 30–45 minutes.

If the researcher or clinician prefers to avoid such lengthy inventories in the assessment of pain, a more practical alternative would be a NRS for each of the common pain experiences in CFS. For instance, a 0 to 100 rating scale could be used to rate the severity of joint pain and diffuse muscle pain. NRSs have consistently demonstrated their validity as pain intensity measures by their positive and significant correlation with other measures of pain intensity and their sensitivities to treatment effects (Karoly & Jensen, 1987).

Measures of Somatic Perception

In an effort to measure symptom perception and symptom amplification in CFS, a few studies have used formal questionnaires.

MODIFIED SOMATIC PERCEPTION QUESTIONNAIRE (MSPQ)

The MSPQ is a 13-item scale that was designed to measure somatic and autonomic symptoms indicative of anxiety and a heightened awareness of body functioning in chronic backache patients (Main, 1983). The scale has been found to be a reliable and valid screening instrument for psychological disturbance in chronic low-back pain. Although the MSPQ has been used in psychological investigations of CFS (e.g., Katon et al., 1991), no validation studies have been done on the MSPQ in populations other than chronic back pain.

PENNEBAKER INVENTORY OF LIMBIC LANGUIDNESS (PILL)

Another symptom perception questionnaire, the PILL (Pennebaker, 1982) measures the frequency of occurrence of 54 common somatic symptoms and sensations (e.g., watering eyes, ringing in the ears, lump in the throat). This inventory has been found to have high reliability and to distinguish individuals who are aware of more bodily symptoms.

High scores on the MPSQ and the PILL may indicate a greater likelihood of psychiatric disorder or symptom amplification in medical patients. However, the ability of any psychometric instrument to make functional–organic distinctions is highly suspect, and in a well-studied population–chronic pain patients—the distinction is essentially meaningless (Tollison & Hinnant, 1996). Furthermore, the concept of symptom amplification is difficult to quantify. Patients who report more somatic symptoms may be accurately perceiving the frequency and intensity of these symptoms or they may be amplifying or overfocusing on them. Somatic perception questionnaires cannot distinguish these possibilities (Barsky, 1996). Alternatively, recent evidence (Aronson & Barrett, 1997) suggests that emotional reactivity (i.e., neuroticism, negative affect) itself may lead to more symptom reporting, independent of somatic sensitivity.

In CFS, which is associated with a number of somatic symptoms, it is difficult for the patient, as well as the clinician, to distinguish appropriate attention to symptoms that may require medical attention from maladaptive overfocusing on symptoms that engenders emotional distress and impairs functioning. Somatic perception inventories may assist the clinician or researcher in identifying the frequency and magnitude of symptom reporting above and beyond the symptoms typically associated with CFS. Because high symptom reporters in CFS are more likely to experience debilitating anxiety and depression (Hickie et al., 1995), somatic perception inventories may help to identify such individuals, who may then be referred for appropriate psychological or medical treatment.

Illness Behavior and Attributions

A concept related to symptom perception is illness behavior. Abnormal illness behavior implies that "the doctor does not believe that the patient's objective pathology entitles him to be placed in a type of sick role he expects for the reasons for which he claims it" (Trigwell et al., 1995, p. 15). Illness attribution is a category of illness behavior that involves patients' beliefs about the causes of their illness.

ILLNESS BEHAVIOR QUESTIONNAIRE (IBQ)

To assess illness behavior, Pilowsky developed the IBQ (Pilowsky, Spence, Cobb, & Katsikitis, 1984) a 62-item self-administered inventory designed to be a multicomponent measure of "the way persons experience and respond to their health status" (p. 123). Seven subscale scores are derived: general hypochondriasis, disease conviction, psychological versus somatic concern, affective inhibition, affective disturbance, denial, and irritability.

Despite the potential usefulness of the IBQ, methodological problems were associated with the procedures used to develop the instrument. Most significantly, the number of individuals who participated in the original scale development was too small for adequate item analysis or the development of specific subscales (Karoly & Jensen, 1987). As a result, subsequent studies have found some but not all of the seven original dimensions (e.g., Main & Waddell, 1987; Pilowski, 1993). The lack of stability of factors and the strong relationship between IBQ scales and measures of emotional discomfort suggest that the IBQ lacks discriminant validity (Karoly & Jensen, 1987). The IBQ in its present form lacks the construct validity required to recommend it as a useful instrument in the evaluation of CFS.

ILLNESS ATTRIBUTION SCALES

Patients' perceptions of the causes of their illness may have important ramifications for long-term outcomes. Several psychological studies of CFS have incorporated illness attribution scales. The scale initially used (Wessely & Powell, 1989) was a single-item, five-point verbal rating that asked participants to what extent they believed their CFS was psychological or physical. The disease conviction subscale of the Illness Behavior Questionnaire (Pilowsky et al., 1984) is a similar measure. Greater physical attribution of the illness has been associated with poorer long-term outcome in a longitudinal study of CFS patients (Wilson et al., 1994) and in outcome assessments of cognitive–behavioral treatment of CFS (S. Butler et al., 1991; Sharpe et al., 1996). These findings may have several interpretations. Greater physical attribution of the illness may indicate (a) denial of the existence of a primary psychological illness (S. Butler et al., 1991; Powell et al., 1990);

(b) an accurate perception of a primary and less controllable biological illness (Friedberg & Krupp, 1994); or (c) rejection of personal responsibility to cope more effectively with the illness, regardless of etiology. Although coping assessments might plausibly provide evidence for one or more of these possibilities, a cross-sectional study of coping in CFS (Ray et al., 1995a) found that illness attributions in CFS patients were unrelated to scores on measures of coping or locus of control beliefs. Clearly, the measurement of illness attribution needs to be refined to better understand its relationship to adjustment and illness outcomes.

FATIGUE-RELATED COGNITIONS SCALE (FRCS)

Dysfunctional beliefs about the symptom of fatigue may be considered a potentially modifiable category of illness behavior. A fatigue belief scale developed in a group of 44 CFS patients and 17 primary depression patients, the FRCS (Appendix D; Friedberg & Krupp, 1994) is a 14-item instrument with a five-point response format that asks patients about their cognitive reactions to fatigue symptoms. Stress-related maladaptive thinking can be identified with this measure. Examples of items include "I think about my fatigue often"; "My fatigue makes me angry"; and "I sometimes think I deserve the fatigue I feel."

The FRCS has shown adequate internal consistency (Cronbach's α = .77). The test differentiates CFS from primary depression in that CFS patients score significantly higher on the scale. In a cognitive–behavioral treatment study of CFS (Friedberg & Krupp, 1994), the FRCS was more sensitive to treatment changes than was the CES-D, the BSI measure of generalized stress, and the FSS. The ability of the FRCS to distinguish CFS from other fatiguing medical illnesses is unknown. Therefore, its psychometric properties have not been fully evaluated. However, the FRCS is an excellent tool for rapid clinical assessment of beliefs about fatigue in CFS patients.

Conclusion

For the researcher, the selection of a mood scale and a functional status measure is essential for psychometric evaluation. The remaining assessment categories reviewed in this chapter, including psychiatric status (global well-being), pain, coping, social support, somatic perception, illness behavior, and illness attribution may or may not be included in CFS investigations, depending on the research questions being asked. The preceding review of specific measures can provide evidence to justify inclusion (or exclusion) of these measures in CFS populations.

For the clinician who is interested in psychometric evaluation, the use of a depression measure such as the BDI and of a functional status measure such as the SF-36 may help to identify important clinical issues and provide a formal basis for outcome assessment when treatment is terminated. Also, the FRCS is a quick way to assess maladaptive thinking about fatigue and target appropriate interventions.

Differential Diagnosis in CFS 7

This chapter can serve as a research-based guide for the CFS diagnostic interview in order to identify and differentiate comorbid psychiatric symptoms associated with clinical depression, somatization disorder, and generalized anxiety disorder. Furthermore, the assessment of stress-related somatic symptoms and personality disorders in CFS patients, as outlined herein, is an important element of clinical evaluation. In the last section of this chapter on differential diagnosis, non-CFS chronic fatigue is distinguished from CFS, as are a variety of overlapping syndromes, including postinfectious Lyme disease, fibromyalgia, multiple chemical sensitivities, and irritable bowel syndrome.

A diagnosis of CFS is appropriately made by a physician who initially rules out other medical conditions that would explain the fatigue symptomatology and then uses the current CDC criteria (Fukuda et al., 1994) to establish a diagnosis of CFS (see Appendix B, "Medical Assessment of CFS"). It should be noted that CFS patients may "doctor shop" for years before a sensitive, CFS-knowledgeable physician is found (Gurwitt et al., 1992). Physicians are often reluctant to diagnose CFS. In an interview study of 20 general practice physicians (Woodward, Broom, & Legge, 1995), 70% were unwilling to make a diagnosis of CFS because of the scientific uncertainty regarding its etiology and a concern that the diagnosis might become a disabling, self-fulfilling prophecy. Patients, by contrast, focused on the sense of validation associated with a disease label and emphasized the detrimental effects of having no explanation for their symptoms.

EXHIBIT 7.1

Symptom Criteria for Melancholic Depression, Based on *DSM-IV*

1. Criteria met for major depression, including loss of pleasure
2. Presence of three or more of the following:
   • Distinct quality of depressed mood
   • Depression worse in the morning
   • Significant weight loss or anorexia
   • Early morning awakening
   • Marked psychomotor agitation or retardation
   • Excessive guilt

DSM-IV = Diagnostic and Statistical Manual of Mental Disorders (4th ed.; American Psychiatric Association, 1994).

The physician may refer the CFS patient to a psychotherapist for treatment of anxiety or depression or to learn coping skills for the illness. The mental health professional can confirm a diagnosis of CFS using the self-report behavioral criteria contained in the current case definition (Fukuda et al., 1994; see Exhibit 1.1, p.11). If the clinician desires a comprehensive symptom assessment, the Symptom Rating Form (see Appendix C) completed by the patient will provide a profile of symptom type and severity. Because CFS symptoms overlap with psychiatric disorders, screening for comorbid psychopathology is important.

Differential Diagnoses: CFS and Depression

The most common co-existing psychological disorder in CFS is depression (Hickie et al., 1990; Kruesi et al., 1989; Lane, Manu, & Matthews, 1991; Millon et al., 1989; Pepper et al., 1993; Wessely & Powell, 1989). In the current CFS case definition (Fukuda et al., 1994), melancholic or psychotic depression is an exclusion criterion. That is, if the patient reports a generalized loss of interest or of enjoyment, or psychotic features, then a diagnosis of CFS is precluded (see Exhibit 7.1).

Preliminary data suggest that generalized loss of interest and enjoyment is unusual in CFS (Friedberg, 1996b). Only 10% of a CFS sample of 36 patients reported the symptom, "I have lost the desire to do things," as compared with 60% of a sample of 44 depressed patients. Also, depressed mood in melancholic depression is usually worse in the morning (*DSM-IV*), whereas in CFS, mood and energy tend to be higher in mid- to late morning (Stone et al., 1994; Wood et al., 1992). However, the exclusion of melancholic and psychotic

EXHIBIT 7.2

Symptoms Common to CFS, Depression, and Generalized Anxiety Disorder

CFS and depression	CFS and generalized anxiety disorder
Fatigue	Fatigue
Sleep disturbance	Sleep disturbance
Poor concentration	Poor concentration
Psychomotor retardation	Irritability
Loss of sexual desire	Restlessness
Nausea	Rapid heartbeat

depression is based on a consensus panel of CFS researchers rather than on empirical data. Therefore, this diagnostic rule should be considered a preliminary guideline.

Nonmelancholic depression and CFS share many symptoms, including persistent fatigue, sleep disturbance, and poor concentration (see Exhibit 7.2). Also, loss of sexual desire and nausea are not uncommon in both depression (Beck, 1967) and CFS (Friedberg, 1995c; Komaroff et al., 1996), even though these symptoms are not listed as formal criteria for either illness. An examination of each of these overlap symptoms will suggest assessment strategies to distinguish the symptomatology of CFS and depression.

FATIGUE

Fatigue is the central feature of CFS. It is severe and persistent, and it could be accurately described as crushing for many affected individuals. In clinical depression, the fatigue reported seldom assumes the prominence that it has in CFS. In primary depression (without CFS), fatigue or loss of energy was reported in 89% of cases in two large sample descriptive studies (Beck, 1967; H. M. Buchwald & Rudick-Davis, 1993). In CFS, severe fatigue was reported in 86–100% of the patients in two large sample investigations (Friedberg et al., 1994; Komaroff et al., 1996). Despite this high level of symptom overlap, the severity and impact of fatigue appears to be much greater in CFS. In a descriptive study of 281 CFS patients (Komaroff et al., 1996) as compared with patients with major depression and MS, severe debilitating fatigue was reported by 100% of CFS patients, 80% of the MS group, and only 28% of patients with major depression. Furthermore, the effect of fatigue on functioning has been found to be significantly greater in CFS than in primary depression, but not significantly different from that in MS patients in comparative studies (S. K. Johnson et al., 1996b; Pepper et al., 1993). Using the terminology of *DSM-IV* depression criteria, fatigue-related psychomotor retardation appears to be much greater in CFS than in depression. Self-rating scales of fatigue severity may be useful in distinguishing the fatigue associated with depression and that associated with CFS (see chap. 5 in this book).

ILLNESS ONSET

Another distinction between CFS and primary depression is the period of time that defines the onset of each illness. In CFS, the illness often develops over several hours to several days (Holmes, Kaplan, Gantz, et al., 1988), whereas depression typically shows a more gradual onset of the symptom complex over weeks or even months (American Psychiatric Association, 1994). Confirming this distinction, a recent comparative study (Komaroff et al., 1996) reported "acute onset" of the illness in 84% of the CFS group, but in 0% of the major depression group. For instance, a depressed person will not become suddenly disabled by fatigue as would a patient with CFS. The difference in the time period of onset between CFS and depression can serve as a rough diagnostic guideline during a clinical evaluation. One 39-year-old patient with CFS described the rapid onset of the illness as follows:

> From time to time I felt persistent fatigue from my job and the stress of the work itself, given the demands that were made on me. The fatigue would always fade away after the weekend, or a vacation. But when I got the illness, the sudden and total exhaustion hit me like a brick. I could hardly get out of bed. Even brushing my teeth was an effort. There's no way I could work. The exhaustion just stayed; it got somewhat better after about a year, but I still couldn't work.

SLEEP DISTURBANCE

Sleep disturbance is a complaint of the vast majority of CFS patients, with insomnia reported by 51% and oversleep by 32% (Friedberg et al., 1994). In large-sample studies of primary depression patients, sleep complaints are common (Beck, 1967; H. M. Buchwald & Rudick-Davis, 1993). A comparative study of CFS, MS, and major depression (Komaroff et al., 1996) found that difficulty falling asleep was reported by 53% of the CFS group but by only 26% of the major depression group. On the other hand, early morning awakening was reported by 58% of the major depression group but by only 19% of the CFS group. In addition, Morriss, Wearden, and Battersby (1997) found that in comparison with primary depression patients, CFS patients ($N = 127$) reported significantly more naps and waking by pain, as well as significantly more difficulty getting to sleep. The investigators concluded that these sleep complaints were either attributable to the lifestyle of CFS patients or seemed inherent to the condition of CFS. Sleep disturbance was unrelated to depression or anxiety.

Polysomnographic studies of CFS patients have documented the existence of sleep disorders, including sleep apnea, hypersomnia, shaky leg syndrome, and narcolepsy in 58–81% of research samples (D. Buchwald et al., 1994; Krupp & Mendelson, 1990; Morriss, Sharpe, Sharpley, & Hawton, 1993). Medical treatment of these sleep disorders may reduce CFS symptomatology, but it does not cure the illness.

The symptom of sleep disturbance may show subtle differences between CFS and depression. Based on clinical observation of CFS patients, we often see a combination of fatigue and a mentally keyed up or "hyper" feeling, such that the individual is exhausted and wanting to sleep but feels mentally wakeful. These paradoxical symptoms during the initial period of sleep onset appear to be much more common in CFS than in depression. The following self-description of a 32-year-old woman with CFS illustrates this phenomenon:

> I'm dragging all day with the fatigue, but I'm able to rest so I can work part-time and handle the job. In the evening, the fatigue and my end-of-the-day tiredness kind of merge together. So I'm ready to go to bed. But, at the same time, I have this hyped up feeling in my head which keeps me from falling asleep. It's like I need a tranquilizer. Eventually, I fall asleep, but it takes a long time and the sleep isn't all that restful.

NEUROCOGNITIVE DIFFICULTIES

Although poor concentration may be a characteristic of both depression and CFS, the deficit appears to be much more profound in CFS. For instance, cognitive problems, including attention and short-term memory deficits, are the principal cause of work disability in some patients. Difficulty concentrating has been reported by 83% of CFS participants in a large sample study (Friedberg, 1995c), whereas 79% of primary depression patients reported difficulty thinking (H. M. Buchwald & Rudick-Davis, 1993; Komaroff et al., 1996). In CFS patients, mental effort to improve concentration may help temporarily, but such efforts may also generate more fatigue and cannot be sustained. The following patient narrative illustrates the profound effects of neurocognitive impairments:

> Since I became ill about a year ago, I get very confused when I drive. I'll forget where I am only a few miles from home on familiar roads. When I'm talking, I'll often forget what I said only seconds before. Now, I have to post reminders all over the

house so I can stay somewhat organized. I know I'm not crazy, but sometimes I think I have "lost" my mind.

A related symptom, distractibility by noise (Friedberg, 1995c), is also frequently reported in CFS. This symptom may contribute to patients' reports that their attention continually drifts. For instance, people with CFS will often state than when walking from one room to another, they will forget why they made the trip. A recent study of noise stress in CFS patients (Beh, 1997) found that CFS participants' performance on a grammatical reasoning task was impaired during exposure to white noise, as compared with healthy controls. Neuropsychological investigations have confirmed deficits in sustained attention in CFS patients (Tiersky, Johnson, Lange, Natelson, & DeLuca, 1997).

LOSS OF SEXUAL DESIRE

In two large sample descriptive studies of CFS patients (Cope et al., 1996; Friedberg et al., 1994), 52–54% reported a loss of sexual desire. The symptom was only minimally correlated ($r = .17$) with the CES-D in the latter study, suggesting that depression was not a cause of the loss of sexual desire. Intuitively, it is not surprising that severe fatigue may deplete sexual desire. In clinical depression, loss of sexual desire has been reported by 58% of a sample of 486 depressed outpatients (Beck, 1967). Although it may not be possible to definitively categorize sexual complaints as CFS or depression related, it is important for the clinician to recognize that reduced libido is not necessarily a manifestation of depression.

JOINT PAIN

Joint pain has been reported by 53% of CFS patients (Friedberg et al., 1994; Komaroff et al., 1996) and by 50% of major depression patients (Komaroff et al., 1996). The high percentage of depressed patients reporting joint pains may be somewhat surprising to mental health professionals. Perhaps this is because joint pain is a secondary concern of the depressed patient, and thus it is not spontaneously reported. Based on these preliminary data (Komaroff et al., 1996), it appears that joint pains cannot be used in differential diagnosis of CFS and depression. Also, medical evaluation of joint pain in CFS often does not reveal definitive signs of inflammation or other markers of disease pathology.

Apart from sensitive clinical observation, many CFS patients can distinguish symptoms of CFS from those of depression. CFS patients are usually familiar with depressive symptoms because of a pre-CFS history of depression or concurrent depression in reaction to their ill-

---

EXHIBIT 7.3

Symptoms More Common in CFS Than in Depression

Prolonged fatigue after exercise
Recurrent sore throat
Painful lymph nodes
Headaches (often pressure-like)
Alcohol intolerance

---

ness. Patients may report, for instance, that they can tell the difference between depression-related fatigue and CFS fatigue. The patient's self-observation of symptoms can assist the clinician in the determination of comorbid diagnoses.

CFS Symptoms Not Common to Depression

Although several symptoms may be shared by CFS and depression, other patient complaints are much more likely to occur in CFS (see Exhibit 7.3).

PROLONGED FATIGUE AFTER EXERCISE

Postexertional malaise or prolonged fatigue after exercise has been reported by 79–87% of CFS research samples (Friedberg et al., 1994; Komaroff et al., 1996) but by only 19% of a sample of major depression patients (Komaroff et al., 1996). Aerobic exercise such as walking, jogging, or swimming, as well as anaerobic activity such as weight lifting, will trigger increased CFS symptoms and even behavioral relapse for many patients (Friedberg et al., 1994). Such exacerbations may not occur until several hours or even a day or two after exercise is completed and may continue for several days or longer (Friedberg et al., 1994). Because a large number of CFS patients engaged in satisfying regular exercise prior to their illness (MacDonald et al., 1996), CFS-related exercise intolerance may trigger emotional sequelae of frustration, anger, and depressed mood. The following case example illustrates how dramatic this change in exercise capacity can be for the individual with CFS. A 30-year-old man described his experience during the initial stages of the illness:

I had been jogging 25 to 30 miles a week for several years. Then, over a three-week period, I began to get intense pressure-like headaches when I was running and prolonged tiredness afterward. As these symptoms worsened, I felt on the verge of collapse and so I had to stop running. After several weeks of no exercise, I felt well enough to start walking. But the same symptoms flared up again. Now I walk short distances two or three days a week, but if I try to do a regular exercise schedule of any kind, my symptoms worsen and I have to stop. This has been a big blow to me, because I love to exercise.

In contrast, individuals with primary depression are less likely to experience symptom flare-ups following exercise. In fact, exercise programs, aerobic or anaerobic, are effective interventions for depression (Martinson, 1987). This differential response to exercise is a key distinction between the two disorders.

COGNITIVE SYMPTOMS

The cognitive symptoms of CFS include dwelling on fatigue sensations, thoughts that one is dying because the symptoms are so severe, and the belief that one has no control over fatigue symptoms (Friedberg, 1995a; Friedberg & Krupp, 1994). A 43-year-old woman with recent CFS described some of these thoughts about her symptoms:

Besides the usual feelings of dragging and tiredness, sometimes I feel like I'm falling apart, almost as if I might die. It's like a profound weakness is overcoming me and my body is just going to break apart because it's too weak to hold together. I don't want to die and I'm not really afraid of dying, but this falling apart feeling can be scary.

The FRCS, a 14-item self-report test described in chapter 6 of this book (see also Appendix D; Friedberg & Krupp, 1994) is designed to assess the frequency of cognitive symptoms in CFS.

In contrast, the cognitive symptoms of depression include thoughts of worthlessness, severe self-criticism, and suicidal or death ideation (American Psychiatric Association, 1994). These types of beliefs, if present, support a diagnosis of depression in CFS. A comparative study of depressive symptomatology in CFS, MS, and clinical depression (S. K. Johnson et al., 1996b) confirmed that self-reproach symptoms such as feelings of failure, guilt, and deserving punishment comprised a significantly greater percentage of total symptoms in the primary depression group as compared with the CFS group.

OTHER SYMPTOMS

The Komaroff et al. (1996) comparative study of CFS, MS, and major depression also revealed other noteworthy differences between CFS and depression. Alcohol intolerance was reported by 60% of the CFS group but by only 21% of the depression sample. Tingling sensations and anorexia were significantly more frequent in the CFS group (55% and 31%, respectively) than in the major depression patients (26% and 5%, respectively). In addition, flu-like symptoms found in CFS (Komaroff et al., 1996), including recurrent sore throat (64%), painful lymph nodes (65%), mild fevers (43%), and headaches (59%) had a low frequency of occurrence (10–22%) in major depression (Komaroff et al., 1996). Finally, nausea was reported by 58% of CFS patients (Friedberg et al., 1994; Komaroff et al., 1996) but by only 16% of depressive patients (Komaroff et al., 1996). Patient reports of one or more of these symptoms will assist in differential diagnosis.

The unusual flu-like symptoms in CFS can be intrusive and debilitating, as the following account from a CFS patient shows:

> If you can imagine what it would be like to be persistently sick with a low-grade flu, then you can begin to understand the illness I have. One particularly annoying symptom: The lymph glands in my neck swell up so that I have a hard time turning my head without increasing the pain and stiffness. Fortunately, I'm still able to work, but I have to focus all my mental energies on what I'm doing; otherwise, I would just succumb to these symptoms and stay home.

CFS and Somatization Disorder

As with depression, the symptoms of somatization disorder show considerable overlap with CFS. The *DSM-IV* criteria for somatization disorder require four pain symptoms, two gastrointestinal symptoms, one sexual symptom, and one pseudoneurological symptom (e.g., impaired coordination or balance, paralysis or localized weakness, difficulty swallowing or lump in the throat). CFS patients may also present with pain, gastrointestinal, sexual, and pseudoneurological symptoms. Because neither condition can be fully explained medically, no diagnostic or laboratory test is available to distinguish CFS from somatization disorder. Therefore, precise clinical differentiation of presenting complaints into CFS and somatization symptoms may not be possible.

How can the clinician distinguish the two disorders? Once again, fatigue is the primary feature of CFS, whereas this symptom is not a listed criterion of somatization disorder. Also, CFS patients typically report a sudden onset of the symptom complex in their late 20s to late 30s (Klonoff, 1992), whereas initial symptoms of somatization disorder begin in adolescence and escalate over several years to full-blown somatization disorder by age 25 (American Psychiatric Association, 1994). To evaluate concurrent somatization disorder in CFS, it is useful to inquire about somatization symptoms prior to the onset of CFS. A history of multiple somatization symptoms that predate CFS onset may suggest the presence of comorbid somatization disorder. However, if somatization-like complaints are associated with the onset of CFS, these complaints may be symptoms of CFS or somatization (S. K. Johnson, DeLuca, & Natelson, 1996a), or they may represent a new stress symptom secondary to CFS, as in the discussion that follows.

CFS and Generalized Anxiety Disorder

Both CFS and generalized anxiety disorder share several symptoms, including fatigue, difficulty concentrating, and sleep disturbance (see Exhibit 7.2). Also, irritability, restlessness, and rapid heartbeat are often characteristic of both disorders, even though they are not on both symptom lists (American Psychiatric Association, 1994; Komaroff et al., 1996). Perhaps the best way to distinguish the two disorders is to focus on the most prominent symptom in each. For generalized anxiety disorder, the primary feature is excessive persistent worry, and in CFS, severe debilitating fatigue. Thus, despite the considerable overlap in symptom criteria, the clinical presentation is quite different. Of course, people with CFS may be persistent worriers as well; therefore, these disorders may co-exist. Comorbid generalized anxiety disorder in CFS has been diagnosed in a significant minority of research samples (e.g., Fischler, Cluydts, Degucht, Kaufman, & Demeirleir, 1997).

CFS and Stress Symptoms

The clinical observation that CFS is a stress-sensitive illness (Friedberg, 1995c) has received empirical support in a comparative study of reactions to a psychological stressor in participants with chronic fatigue, anxiety or depressive disorders, or muscular dystrophy (Wood et al., 1994). The chronic fatigue group, who met Oxford (British) criteria for CFS (see Appendix A; Sharpe et al., 1991), evidenced the largest increase in self-rated psychological and physical symptoms in reaction

TABLE 7.1

Stress–Symptom Log

Day/Time	Event	Stress rating	Fatigue rating
Tuesday			
9:30 a.m.	Argued with husband	6	6
3:00 p.m.	Kids were screaming	5	7
8:00 p.m.	Walked around the block	5	8

Note: 0 = *least*; 10 = *most*.

to a timed anagram task. The stress generated by such mental effort is one of the most debilitating aspects of CFS, as the following patient narrative illustrates:

> Whenever I try to read something, I can only concentrate on the text for a few minutes. Then I start to get confused and mentally clouded. I have to put down the book or article and just rest from the "exertion" of reading. I get tired just from a few minutes of reading! Before I became ill, I was an avid reader of books, newspapers, magazines, you name it. Now I have to slowly pace my reading so I don't get too tired.

There are at least two ways that stress may directly increase symptoms in CFS patients. First, any stressor—physical or emotional—may increase CFS symptoms (Friedberg et al., 1994; Wood et al., 1994). The most frequently endorsed relapse triggers in CFS in a descriptive study of 313 participants with CFS (Friedberg et al., 1994) were physical exertion (97%), exercise (85%), and emotional stress (80%). Second, stress may trigger somatic reactions other than CFS symptoms. These types of stress reactions may include anxiety- or anger-related symptoms such as stomach upset, rapid heartbeat, or muscular tension.

The clinician can help the patient to become aware of these stress–symptom connections and use this information to design treatment interventions. A stress–symptom log (see Table 7.1) wherein the patient enters daily numerical ratings of stress and symptom levels (Lazarus, 1976) will reveal how physical and emotional stressors affect symptom severity. The daily charting is especially useful for (a) persistent but low-level stressors that may worsen symptoms without the patient's awareness and (b) delayed symptom exacerbations in response to stressors that may not occur until 1 or 2 days after the stress exposure. For instance, fear about new symptoms is a common stress reaction in early CFS, as the symptom complex unfolds over many months (Friedberg, 1995c). As new symptoms arise, the patient may wonder if they are premonitory signals of a more serious illness, a part of the CFS, or reactions to stress. As the patient recognizes stress–symptom associations, he or she is less likely to become worried about the meaning of any new symptom.

To further evaluate stress symptoms, the clinician may ask, (a) "How do you react to stress now?" and (b) "How did you react to stress before you were ill?" As the therapist identifies somatic stress reactions, the patient can be reassured that these stress responses may occur more frequently and with greater intensity because of the increased psychological and physical reactivity associated with CFS (Wood et al., 1994). Then stress reduction techniques (see chap. 9 in this book) can be applied to moderate symptom flare-ups and stress reactions to them. Identifying stress symptoms will also assist in diagnosing co-existing psychological disorders.

Axis II Disorders in CFS

Studies of personality disorders in CFS have found significantly fewer Axis II diagnoses in CFS, compared with primary depression groups (S. K. Johnson et al., 1996c; Pepper et al., 1993), and no significant differences in frequency or type of Axis II diagnoses between patients with CFS and MS (S. K. Johnson et al., 1996c; Pepper et al., 1993). The majority of the Axis II disorders in the S. K. Johnson et al. (1996c) report were found in CFS participants with concurrent depressive disorder. The most frequently diagnosed Axis II disorders have been compulsive personality (Pepper et al., 1993) and histrionic personality (S. K. Johnson et al., 1996c). The compulsive personality may be related to the premorbid overachievement lifestyles of many individuals with CFS (N. C. Ware, 1993).

It should be noted that a substantial number of individuals with CFS (22–76% of research samples in psychodiagnostic studies [Friedberg, 1996a]) had no diagnosable psychiatric disorder. However, these nonpsychiatric CFS patients may well have treatable stress problems and coping difficulties, as might be associated with any chronic disabling condition.

Structured Psychodiagnostic Evaluation

Given the problems described above in distinguishing CFS and psychiatric symptoms, the use of structured psychodiagnostic interviews may offer a higher level of standardization and precision for diagnostic classification. On the other hand, the decision rules for the specific structured interview may also bias diagnostic assignment. This section summarizes the research on the use of structured clinical interviews and may be especially useful for researchers who incorporate diagnostic interviews in their study designs.

The Diagnostic Interview Schedule (DIS), a structured psychiatric instrument designed for use in community surveys (Robins & Regier, 1991), has frequently been used to assess psychiatric comorbidity in CFS samples. Unfortunately, this instrument was not designed for use with medically ill populations. In addition, each CFS investigator may administer this instrument somewhat differently.

The CDC has significantly modified both the administration and scoring of this instrument for CFS evaluation (Lea Steele, personal communication, August 1, 1993). For example, in the Somatization section, question D4—a required question on the original DIS—has been left out of the modified DIS. Question D4 was as an integral part of the Panic Disorder section; paraphrased, it reads, "Were you ever bothered by [somatization-type symptoms] at any time other than when you were having one of these spells [panic attacks]?" If the respondent answers "yes" to this question, he or she might meet criteria for both Somatization Disorder and Panic Disorder. If the respondent answers "no," however, he or she is eligible to meet the criteria only for Panic Disorder. This is an important question in distinguishing between respondents with panic disorder only, those with somatization disorder only, and those with both panic disorder and somatization disorder. By excluding a question similar to D4, the number of respondents with *DSM-III-R* somatization disorder may be overestimated, given that many panic disorder symptoms may be mistaken as somatization disorder symptoms. Because somatization symptoms in CFS are difficult to identify and may be overestimated (S. K. Johnson et al., 1996a), the elimination of the above question on the DIS may further inflate the frequency of erroneous somatization diagnoses.

In addition, research teams using the DIS are employing different decision rules in scoring responses; these decision rules determine whether symptoms are viewed as resulting from medical illness or from psychiatric disorders. For example, if a respondent mentions that a symptom on the DIS (e.g., pains in arms or legs) was due to a medical problem that was diagnosed by a physician, DIS rules dictate that this problem should not be counted as a psychiatric problem. On the other hand, if the respondent had no contact with a doctor, yet still claims that the symptom was the result of a physical illness or injury, the DIS directions dictate that the administrator should take the respondent's word for it (but if the interviewer believes that the respondent is probably mistaken, an editor might later recode the response to indicate a psychiatric problem). Many CFS researchers are not following these directions but are coding both responses as psychiatric problems, thus increasing the likelihood of psychiatric comorbidity.

An additional problem with the DIS is that the score that the participant receives heavily depends on the opinion of any previously consulted physician. If the physician had attributed the patient's symptoms to a nervous or psychiatric disorder, the patient automatically receives a score counting toward a psychiatric diagnosis, whether or not the patient agrees with the physician. Also, if several physicians diagnosed a patient as having a medical disorder, but only one arrived at the diagnosis of a nervous disorder, the item would be scored to count toward a psychiatric diagnosis. Many physicians still do not accept CFS as a legitimate medical disorder. Thus it is possible that patients would have encountered at least one physician who misdiagnosed their medical complaints as psychiatric or nervous disorders. Such misidentification would increase the likelihood that people with CFS would receive unwarranted psychiatric diagnoses on a structured interview. Finally, if the patient had not consulted a physician and could not offer a specific cause for a symptom, the symptom would receive a psychiatric score, provided that it was not due to the patient's ingestion of alcohol or prescribed or nonprescribed drugs or to the presence of physical illness or injury, as determined by the interviewer.

COMPARATIVE PSYCHODIAGNOSTIC STUDIES

Many of the CFS minor symptoms are contained within *DSM-IV* categories. Thus, a person with CFS might specify a large number of physical problems caused by the illness, although these physical complaints would also make the person eligible for a diagnosis of depression or somatization disorder. When Demitrack (1993) used restrictive criteria for psychodiagnosis that excluded symptoms attributable to CFS, 6 of 30 CFS patients had a lifetime history of major depression, but when criteria were used that included all symptoms as psychiatrically relevant, 12 of 30 CFS patients had a lifetime history of major depressive illness. A similar finding has been reported for somatization disorder in CFS. S. K. Johnson et al. (1996a) compared CFS patients with those with MS, those with depression, and a healthy control group. Changing the attribution of somatization symptoms from a psychiatric to a physical one dramatically affected the rates of diagnosis of somatization in the CFS group; rates ranged from 0 to 98%, depending on whether or not CFS symptoms were coded as a physical illness. Several other investigators have found similar discrepancies in comparing these different scoring systems (Abbey, 1993).

In contrast to the rigid interview structure of the DIS, the Structured Clinical Interview for *DSM-III-R* (SCID; Robins, Helzer, Cottler, & Goldring, 1989) uses open-ended questions and all potential sources of information to encourage a thorough description of the problems by the interviewer, who must be a specifically trained clinician. The SCID also assesses information about subthreshold symptoms, permitting an analysis of individuals who approach but do not actually meet criteria for specific psychiatric diagnoses. The SCID was the instrument used on a sample of CFS patients by Hickie et al., (1990), who found the premorbid prevalence of major depressive disorder to be 12.5%, and overall psychiatric disorders to be 24.5%, rates which are no higher than general community estimates. Lloyd et al., (1990) also used the SCID and found a past prevalence of major depressive disorders in 21% of patients with CFS, and a past prevalence of overall psychiatric disorders in 39%. These rates are higher than reported in Hickie et al., (1990), but not nearly as high as psychiatric disorder prevalence reported in studies of CFS using the DIS.

A recent study by Taylor and Jason (in press) attempted to resolve this discrepancy in psychiatric rates between the DIS and the SCID by administering both interviews to a CFS sample and then comparing the results. Of 18 individuals diagnosed with CFS, 50% of the sample received at least one current Axis I psychiatric diagnosis when the DIS was used; however, only 22% received such a diagnosis when the SCID was used. These findings suggest that the discrepant psychiatric rates reported in past studies might have been due in part to the psychiatric instrument that was used.

RESEARCH STRATEGIES TO STUDY DEPRESSION IN CFS

Several CFS researchers have recommended a more refined analysis of depression symptoms in order to better differentiate depression and CFS. Ray (1991) proposed that the assessment of depression in CFS be carried out with multidimensional constructs. Specifically, symptoms of depression could be grouped into three categories: affective (i.e., irritability, dysphoric mood, anhedonia), cognitive (i.e., negative interpretations of themselves and the world), and somatic (i.e., alterations in weight, sleep patterns, increased fatigability, dry mouth, constipation, and headaches). Brickman and Fins (1993) suggested that focusing on the affective and cognitive components of CFS may allow investigators to reduce the possible confounding effects of somatic symptoms. For instance, individuals with depressive disorders often experience anhedonia (a loss of pleasure) and feelings of worthlessness, symptoms that are usually not experienced by individuals with CFS unless they have comorbid depression.

In support of this distinction between cognitive and somatic symptoms, S. K. Johnson et al. (1996b) found that patients with CFS reported significantly fewer self-reproach symptoms and a significantly higher percentage of somatic symptoms than did a sample diagnosed with primary depression. With regard to loss of pleasure, individuals with CFS (Wessely & Powell, 1989) scored between those with neuromuscular disorders and those with affective disorders on the Hospital Anxiety and Depression Scale, a measure devised for physically ill patients with items for depression based on the anhedonic state. Thus, patients with CFS experienced less pleasure than neuromuscular patients and more pleasure than those with depression. In addition, as previously discussed, mood level in people who are depressed is lowest in the morning, although it may rise during the day. In people with CFS, energy and mood are highest in the mid-morning (Wood et al., 1992).

We believe that structured psychiatric interviews for medical patients in general, and CFS patients in particular, must be responsive to psychodiagnostic research and informed clinical observation, as outlined above, in order to fulfill their objectives as valid measures of psychiatric disorders.

Non-CFS Chronic Fatigue

Some patients will report persistent fatigue and exhaustion related to concurrent psychosocial factors (Jason, Taylor, et al., 1995). Careful assessment of these individuals reveals that they do not have CFS. At least two different types of clinical presentations are associated with (non-CFS) chronic fatigue:

ACTIVITY-INDUCED CHRONIC FATIGUE

Individuals in this category who report ongoing fatigue are leading hectic lifestyles with a variety of obligations and inadequate time for sleep, rest, and relaxation. However, a vacation or a reduction in personal responsibilities will allow fatigue symptoms to resolve and normal energy levels and functioning to return. Clearly, psychological interventions may be appropriate for such individuals, but without the complications associated with CFS. A sociological monograph (Schor, 1991) that tracked work and recreation habits in the

United States found that Americans worked more and enjoyed less leisure time in the 1990s compared with the 1970s. The study suggested that generalized overwork may lead to more stress-related disorders. Thus, activity-induced chronic fatigue may be a more common phenomenon in today's work-focused culture.

CHRONIC FATIGUE ASSOCIATED WITH LIFE TRANSITION

Patients in this category may be undergoing a significant life change (e.g. termination of a relationship, change of job, death in the family) that engenders a temporary emotional reaction experienced predominantly as fatigue. When the emotional sequelae associated with the life transition are resolved, a return to precrisis functioning occurs. Recovery from life transition chronic fatigue typically occurs in less than the 6 months required by the case criteria for CFS. Of course, psychotherapy may be initiated for the life change issues.

In contrast to non-CFS fatigue, the fatigue in CFS is severe and persistent even in the absence of any significant activity (Fukuda et al., 1994). Mild exertion will increase the fatigue symptoms, but sleep and rest will not restore normal energy levels. Careful questioning of the client as suggested by the guidelines above will help to differentiate CFS from stress-induced chronic fatigue.

Syndromes That Overlap With CFS

Many of the symptoms associated with CFS are also characteristic of other poorly understood illness conditions, including postinfectious Lyme disease, fibromyalgia, multiple chemical sensitivities, and irritable bowel syndrome. Because the CFS patient may report one or more of these overlap syndromes, it is important for the treating clinician to recognize the specific symptomatic presentation. In the absence of definitive diagnostic markers or laboratory tests to distinguish these conditions, clinical diagnosis is largely based on self-report symptoms and behavioral criteria. A recent study of functional somatic distress (Robbins, Kirmayer, & Hemami, 1997), using latent variable models in a sample of 686 family medicine patients, tentatively confirmed that CFS, fibromyalgia, and irritable bowel syndrome represent discrete entities.

POSTINFECTIOUS LYME DISEASE

Lyme disease, a rheumatological condition, is caused by an infectious spirochete, *Borrelia burgdorferi* (Nocton & Steere, 1995). The disease is contracted through a tick bite, which causes a rash in 40–50% of cases. The initial symptoms include joint pain and swelling, headaches, cognitive difficulties, and fatigue. Early treatment with antibiotics is curative in most cases (Nocton & Steere, 1995). However, some cases of treated Lyme disease will result in a temporary remission of symptoms, followed by a resurgence of symptoms without evidence of continuing Lyme infection. The clinical presentation of the postinfectious Lyme patient is indistinguishable from CFS (Sigal, 1994). It is not clear why most Lyme patients completely recover while a minority remain symptomatic and sometimes disabled (Sigal, 1994). For the behavioral clinician, the approach to diagnosis and treatment of post-Lyme CFS is essentially identical to that taken with non-Lyme CFS.

FIBROMYALGIA

Fibromyalgia (FM) is a common rheumatologic ailment characterized by chronic generalized muscle pain, fatigue, and disrupted sleep. Proposed criteria for the diagnosis of FM require widespread muscular pain in conjunction with tenderness at a minimum number of tender points (Wolfe, Smythe, Yunus, Bennett, & Bombardier, 1990). FM is often associated with headache, irritable bowel syndrome, and interstitial cystitis. It occurs most commonly in women and may follow an acute medical illness, a traumatic injury, or surgery (Greenfield, Fitzcharles, & Esdaile, 1992; Waylonis & Perkins, 1994). Several previous studies have suggested that CFS and FM are similar if not identical conditions (D. Buchwald, 1996; Goldenberg, 1988; Goldenberg, Simms, Geiger, & Komaroff, 1990).

In a multigroup study (D. Buchwald & Garrity, 1994), patients with CFS, FM, and multiple chemical sensitivities were compared on symptom criteria. Seventy percent of patients with FM met criteria for CFS. In a comparison of specific symptoms, no significant differences were found in symptom prevalence between CFS and FM, except for painful lymph nodes, which were significantly more frequent in the FM group (67%) compared with the CFS group (27%). In a subsequent comparative study of chronic fatigue, CFS, and FM (Bombardier & Buchwald, 1996), patients diagnosed with both CFS and FM were substantially more disabled than patients with either condition alone. Schaefer (1995) found, in a comparison of FM and CFS patients, that women with CFS reported significantly more trouble staying asleep than women with FM, although both groups had high levels of overall sleep disturbance.

A cognitive–behavioral treatment study of FM (Nielson, Walker, & McCain, 1992) and a follow-up report (K. P. White & Nielson, 1995) found immediate and sustained improvements 30 months post-treatment in worry, observed pain behavior, and control over pain. For the CFS patient with concurrent FM, pain symptoms may become a primary target for psychological interventions. The cognitive–behavioral treatments described in subsequent chapters in this book may be adapted for pain symptoms as well.

MULTIPLE CHEMICAL SENSITIVITIES

Unlike CFS and FM, there are no universally agreed on criteria for multiple chemical sensitivities (MCS). One commonly used case definition (Cullen, 1987) describes it as an acquired disorder triggered by exposure to diverse chemicals at doses far below those documented to cause adverse affect in humans. Symptoms are recurrent, involve many organ systems, and are elicited by exposure to the offending chemical compounds. However, individuals with MCS are often unaware of or unable to identify the reaction-eliciting chemicals (I. Bell, 1996). Typical symptoms include those of skin or mucous membrane irritation, fatigue, myalgias, fevers, and neurocognitive dysfunction. In the D. Buchwald and Garrity (1994) study cited earlier, 30% of those individuals with MCS met criteria for CFS. Self-reported high levels of reactivity to chemical exposures have also been found in CFS patients in comparison with healthy controls (Friedberg et al., 1994).

A principal treatment modality for MCS involves minimizing exposure to the offending chemicals using such tactics as eliminating carpeting, pesticides, and cleaning agents from the home and avoiding perfume, tobacco smoke, and other presumably toxic substances. Data on the efficacy of these environmental alterations is lacking, although a recent survey of patients with MCS, 41% of whom had comorbid CFS, reported on the efficacy of a number of interventions for MCS (see chap. 8 in this book). For the CFS patient with MCS, the identification of chemical sensitivities and attempts to eliminate triggering substances may lead to symptom reductions in some patients. For further information on MCS, we recommend L. Lawson's *Staying Well in a Toxic World* (1993).

IRRITABLE BOWEL SYNDROME

Irritable bowel syndrome (IBS), a functional gastrointestinal disorder, is a symptom-based diagnosis requiring at least 3 months of continuous or recurrent symptoms of abdominal pain or discomfort associated with changes in bowel habits or stool characteristics (Drossman &

Thompson, 1992). A high incidence of comorbid psychiatric disorders in irritable bowel syndrome has been reported (Lydiard, Fossey, Marsh, & Ballenger, 1993). In one large sample study of CFS (Friedberg et al., 1994), 67% of 285 long-term CFS patients reported having IBS. By comparison, IBS has been reported to occur in 8–17% of the general population (Drossman & Thompson, 1992). At least six cognitive–behavioral treatment studies have shown favorable results in the treatment of IBS (Drossman, 1995). The cognitive–behavioral techniques described in chapter 9 in this book, especially relaxation training, may be helpful in the treatment of comorbid IBS.

Conclusion

This chapter amply illustrates the difficulties in distinguishing CFS symptoms from symptoms of depression, somatization, and anxiety disorders. Also, the influence of stress and personality disorders on CFS are important clinical issues in the assessment and treatment of the illness. Overlap syndromes that may co-occur with CFS, including postinfectious Lyme disease, FM, MCS, and irritable bowel syndrome may further complicate assessment with the presentation of additional disabling symptoms. A full appreciation of the complex symptom dimensions of CFS and related conditions will allow the clinician and the researcher to construct appropriate, data-based assessments and interventions.

TREATMENT

Medical and
Alternative Therapies

8

No effective treatment or cure is yet available for CFS. However, promising new treatments have been reported. The inability of conventional medicine to help CFS sufferers, combined with the skepticism of many physicians about the existence of the illness have led many patients to seek alternative therapies (Ax, Gregg, & Jones, 1997; Denz-Penhey & Murdoch, 1993). In this chapter, we present studies of pharmacological and alternative therapies for CFS, followed by patients' ratings of treatment effectiveness.

Pharmacological Treatment

ANTIVIRAL AND IMMUNOMODULATORY DRUGS

Few studies of pharmacological intervention for CFS have been reported. Because CFS patients often report prominent flu-like symptoms, a viral illness was initially suspected. A double-blind placebo controlled study of Acyclovir, an antiviral agent chosen on the basis of data linking the syndrome to the Epstein-Barr virus, showed no significant differences between placebo and drug conditions in CFS patients (Straus, Dale, Tobi, et al., 1988). As no virus or other identified pathogen was consistently associated with CFS in subsequent studies, an immune system defect was proposed to account for chronic fatigue symptoms. Consequently, pharmacological treatments for immune dysfunction were explored.

An immune system modulator, mismatched double-stranded RNA (Ampligen), significantly improved functional status and reduced symptoms in severely disabled CFS patients in a double-blind placebo controlled study (Strayer et al., 1994). A subsequent clinical study of Ampligen (Strayer, Carter, Strauss, Brodsky, & Suhadolnik, 1995) in 15 severely disabled CFS patients found sustained improvements over a 48-week period in functional status, cognitive complaints, and exercise tolerance. Also, reductions were evidenced in human herpesvirus-6, a herpesvirus that may play a role in CFS pathogenesis (Strayer et al., 1995).

The maker of Ampligen received FDA approval in the spring of 1997 to begin an open clinical trial for severely disabled CFS patients (*CFIDS* News, 1997). Only 11 US physicians are prescribing Ampligen for their CFS patients under an agreement with the manufacturer, although a spokesman for the company recently told us that they hope to have 50 treating physicians in about a year. Ampligen is an expensive treatment, carrying a cost of $6,900–$15,000 for a standard 6-month protocol, depending on the number of infusions. The treatment is recommended for those patients with sudden onset of symptoms who have cognitive deficits. However, long-term follow-up data for those who have completed Ampligen treatment is still limited.

Other immune modulators, including immunoglobulin (Vollmer-Conna et al., 1997), dialyzable leukocyte (transfer factor), gamma globulin, interferons, and corticosteriods have not proved efficacious for CFS patients (Blondel-Hill & Shafran, 1993), although a recent controlled trial of alpha interferon treatment (See & Tilles, 1996) significantly improved quality of life scores in the subset of CFS patients with natural killer-cell dysfunction.

ANTIDEPRESSANT MEDICATIONS

Disturbances in brain neurochemistry shared by CFS and major depression may serve as a basis for the effectiveness of some antidepressants in CFS (Goodnick & Sandoval, 1993), although a therapeutic response may occur at doses lower than those used in major depression (e.g., Amitriptyline, 10–75 mg/day). A few case reports describe beneficial antidepressant intervention in CFS. For instance, Nortriptyline, a tricyclic antidepressant (TCA) was tested in a single-case double-blind study in the treatment of CFS (Goodnick & Sandoval, 1993). A 60-mg-per-day dose significantly reduced Beck depression scores and CFS symptom scores. In controlled trials, TCAs have produced symptom improvements in fibromyalgia, an illness closely related to CFS (Blondel-Hill & Shafran, 1993). The clinically observed efficacy of subclinical doses of TCAs in CFS suggests that symptom reduction is not based on an antidepressant effect. However, CFS patients may experience significant side effects, including sedation and fatigue exacerbation, from first-generation TCAs (Lynch, Seth, & Montgomery, 1990).

Alternatively, the use of fluoxetine (Prozac), an antidepressant with fewer sedative and autonomic nervous system side effects, has been suggested for CFS patients (Lynch et al., 1990). Despite encouraging results from two preliminary case series using fluoxetine in CFS patients (Goodnick & Sandoval, 1993), a recent double-blind placebo controlled trial of the drug (20 mg/day) in CFS patients (Vercoulen, Swanink, Zitman, et al., 1996) showed no beneficial effect on any characteristic of CFS, including fatigue severity, depression, functional limitations, sleep disturbance, and cognitive functioning. As no dose–response relationship has been established for fluoxetine (Gram, 1994), it is not clear that higher dosages would have improved outcome. Given that 44.7% of the sample met criteria for major depression, it is surprising that depression symptoms were not ameliorated by fluoxetine. The authors suggested that the selective seratonin re-uptake blocking mechanism of fluoxetine is not effective in CFS because depressed CFS patients do not show disturbed seratonin processes (Yatham et al., 1995).

Finally, an open trial of the antidepressant drug moclobemide, a monoamine oxidase inhibitor, on 49 patients with CFS (P. D. White & Cleary, 1997) resulted in significant but small reductions in fatigue, depression, anxiety, and somatic amplification, as well as modest overall improvement. The greatest improvement occurred in those individuals who had a comorbid major depressive illness. The authors concluded that moclobemide may be beneficial for CFS patients with comorbid depressive illness.

BLOOD PRESSURE MEDICATIONS

The association between low blood pressure, fatigue, and headaches provided the rationale for a study of neurally mediated hypotension in CFS patients (Bou-Holaigah, Rowe, Kan, & Calkins, 1995). This condition occurs when the patient changes position to upright but the central nervous system misinterprets the positional change and sends a message to the heart to slow down and lower the blood pressure. These responses are directly opposite to what the body needs. The symptoms produced include dizziness, fainting, and chronic fatigue. The Bou-Holaigah et al. (1995) study compared the clinical symptoms and blood pressure response evoked by diagnostic testing (i.e., tilt table test) in healthy individuals and patients with CFS. An abnormal blood pressure response was observed in 22 of 23 CFS patients but in only 4 of 14 controls. Nine out of 19 patients reported complete, or nearly complete, resolution of CFS symptoms when treated with blood pressure medications. The authors concluded that neurally mediated hypotension can be effectively treated in a subset of CFS patients. These findings await replication in a placebo controlled study.

Although medications (most commonly low-dosage tranquilizers and antidepressants) may prove efficacious for some patients in the management of anxiety and depression as well as in the management of the CFS symptoms of sleep disturbance, headache and body pain, it should be noted that CFS patients are often sensitive even to sub-clinical doses of prescribed drugs (Francis, 1990; Gurwitt et al., 1992) and may report adverse reactions (Twemlow et al., 1997). Patients should be directed to physicians who are both knowledgeable about the syndrome and sensitive to patient complaints. Local CFS support group organizations can usually offer recommendations.

Alternative Therapies for CFS

CFS patients, especially those who are severely disabled, may be desperate to try any potential treatment for their illness, even though newly touted therapies for the illness are often experimental at best or entirely untested at worst. Perhaps the most frequently tried nonconventional therapy is vitamin, mineral, and amino acid supplementation. Although a majority of CFS individuals report having tried self-directed or professionally prescribed vitamin therapies (Friedberg et al., 1994), few studies of dietary intervention have been published. A preliminary report on vitamin C infusions for a large sample of CFS patients (Kodama, Kodama, & Murakami, 1996) suggests that this treatment may be helpful. On the other hand, a treatment once advocated in southern California—injections of liver extract containing folic acid and cyanocobalamin—was found to be ineffective as a treatment for CFS in a double-blind placebo controlled study (Kaslow, Rucker, & Onishi, 1989).

Another approach to dietary intervention is based on magnesium supplementation. Initial data suggesting that CFS individuals have lower red blood cell magnesium than do healthy controls (Cox, Campbell, & Dowson, 1991) provided the empirical basis for a randomized double-blind placebo controlled study of intramuscular magnesium sulphate injections in 32 patients with CFS. Significant improvements in energy, diminished pain, and reduced "emotional reactions" were found in the treatment group but not in the placebo condition. Outcome was determined by questionnaire without physiological measures or follow-up data. Replication of these findings has not been reported.

A third type of dietary treatment is based on the hypothesis that disordered metabolism of fatty acids might play a role in CFS (Behan, Behan, & Horrobin, 1990). The abnormal fatigability and muscle pain complaints in CFS are similar to the symptoms of carnitine (an essential fatty acid) deficiency (Rebouche & Engel, 1983). The Behan research team cited evidence for persistently low levels of serum fatty acids following acute infections such as Epstein-Barr virus. These fatty acids may remain low and correlate with the common experience of postinfectious physical malaise. A prospective, randomized double-blind placebo controlled treatment study (Behan et al., 1990) using essential fatty acids (e.g., fish oil and primrose oil), reported beneficial effects for CFS patients compared with the placebo group. Significant declines in reported muscle pain were found at treatment termination, and a 3-month follow-up revealed significant improvements in questionnaire scores for fatigue, malaise, dizziness, concentration, and depression. Overall, 74% reported improvements in the treatment condition, whereas only 23% were improved in the placebo condition. No functional status assessment was reported.

A recent study comparing carnitine and amantadine (a drug used for the treatment of fatigue in MS) for CFS patients in a crossover design (Plioplys & Plioplys, 1997) found statistically significant improvements in 12 of the 18 studied parameters after 8 weeks of treatment. Improvements were noted on indices of CFS severity and impairment, depression (BDI), and generalized distress (SCL-90-R). No in vivo measures, such as return to work, were reported. Amantadine was poorly tolerated by patients, and no significant improvements were found with this drug. Finally, an unpublished controlled study of essential fatty acids showed no differences between a CFS treated group and a placebo condition (McBride & McCluskey, 1991). Given the positive results for the dietary intervention of essential fatty acids in two out of three studies, it appears that further investigation is warranted.

Finally, specific interventions for a controversial condition called "candida hypersensitivity syndrome" (CHS) have been advocated for CFS, which shares many symptoms with CHS. CHS purportedly is caused by a systemic overgrowth of *Candida albicans*, a yeast-like fungus that is a normal commensal in the human gut (Blondel-Hill & Shafran, 1993). Candida can act as a systemic pathogen in the immunosuppressed (e.g., HIV-infected patients) or may cause localized candidiasis in the mouth or genitalia following broad-spectrum antibiotics, which disrupt the normal bacterial flora (McBride & McCluskey, 1991).

Many alternative health practitioners (e.g., clinical ecologists, naturopaths) believe that candida overgrowth is a maintenance factor in CFS and that candida eradication will promote recovery. The condition is treated with special diets and antifungal medications. A search of Medline revealed no studies of dietary intervention for CHS, although 27% of CFS participants in one study (Friedberg et al., 1994) retrospectively reported moderate to major illness improvements on an "anti-yeast" diet.

A lengthy list of unconventional treatments for CFS have been advocated by alternative health practitioners, including herbal remedies, homeopathy, colonic irrigation, hydrotherapy, chelation, acupuncture, blue/green algae, magnets, and therapeutic touch. In general, no published data (other than the survey findings below) are available to adjudge the efficacy of these interventions for CFS. However, two studies of alternative treatments merit consideration. A randomized controlled trial ($N = 20$) of massage therapy as compared with an attention control condition (sham transcutaneous electrical nerve stimulation [TENS]) for patients with CFS showed significant improvements in generalized distress, sleep, anxiety, pain, depression, fatigue, and somatic symptoms on self-report measures (Field et al., 1997). The massage group, as compared with the sham TENS condition, also evidenced significant decreases in the stress-related hormone, cortisol. Clearly, the stress-reducing effects of massage may be beneficial to the highly stressed population of CFS patients.

Another alternative approach to CFS treatment, electroencephalographic (EEG) biofeedback, is supported by a preliminary case study (James & Folen, 1996). These authors stated that CFS patients have an atypical EEG, comprising a high-amplitude delta (<4 Hz) brainwave activity and an abnormally low-amplitude beta (13–25 Hz) activity. The treatment involved 4 days a week of 40–45 minute neuro-biofeedback sessions for 3 months. Test results on selected subtests of the Wechsler Adult Intelligence Scale–Revised (WAIS-R), supported by clinical findings, revealed improvements in the patient's cognitive abilities, functional skill level, and quality of life. No follow-up data were reported.

Patient Ratings of Treatment Effectiveness

Patient ratings of treatment efficacy based on their personal experience with specific therapies have appeared in a descriptive study of CFS

TABLE 8.1

Treatment Effectiveness Rated by Individuals With CFS

N[a]	Treatment tried	Moderate to major improvement (%)	Worsened condition (%)
3	Ampligen	100	0
186	Anti-allergy diet	32	<1
249	Antidepressant medications	28	31
183	Anti-yeast diet	27	5
133	Stress reduction/biofeedback	26	<1
114	IV vitamins/injections	26	4
180	Physical therapy/massage	26	16
109	Acupuncture	25	10
60	Kutapressin	25	12
65	Macrobiotic diet	23	15
184	Psychotherapy	19	7
283	Vitamin/mineral/amino acid therapy	18	5
127	Allergy shots	17	27
129	Homeopathy	16	12
112	Tagamet or other H2 blocker	16	13
80	Malic acid	16	14
76	Gamma globulin	16	20
38	IV antibiotics	16	39
207	Anti-inflammatory drugs	14	16
81	Antiviral drugs	14	19
195	Oral antibiotics	14	36
55	Removal of amalgam fillings	13	9
55	Magnesium injections	13	11
184	Herbal remedies	13	15
161	Co-enzyme Q10	11	13
10	Transfer factor	10	30
44	Nitroglycerin	9	25
26	Alpha/Beta Interferon	8	23
17	Chelation therapy	6	12

Note: From *Coping With Chronic Fatigue Syndrome: Nine Things You Can Do* (pp. 23–24) by F. Friedberg, 1995, Oakland, CA: New Harbinger. Copyright 1995 by New Harbinger Publications. Reprinted with permission.
[a]Sample sizes ≥ 25 yield more reliable results.

(Friedberg et al., 1994). Table 8.1 shows CFS patient rankings of treatment effectiveness for 29 listed medical and alternative therapies (Friedberg et al., 1994) Two relatively benign interventions, anti-allergy diet and anti-yeast diet, were more highly rated than were the vast majority of pharmacologic therapies. Unfortunately, systematic dietary interventions are usually not prescribed by clinical physicians, despite growing evidence of the important role of dietary factors in the pathogenesis of major chronic illnesses such as heart disease and

FIGURE 8.1

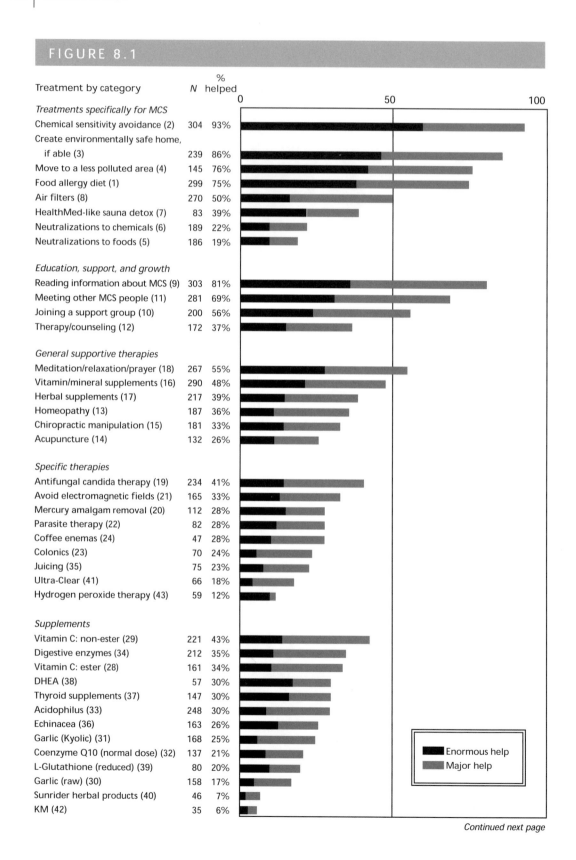

Treatment by category — N — % helped

Treatments specifically for MCS
Treatment	N	% helped
Chemical sensitivity avoidance (2)	304	93%
Create environmentally safe home, if able (3)	239	86%
Move to a less polluted area (4)	145	76%
Food allergy diet (1)	299	75%
Air filters (8)	270	50%
HealthMed-like sauna detox (7)	83	39%
Neutralizations to chemicals (6)	189	22%
Neutralizations to foods (5)	186	19%

Education, support, and growth
Treatment	N	% helped
Reading information about MCS (9)	303	81%
Meeting other MCS people (11)	281	69%
Joining a support group (10)	200	56%
Therapy/counseling (12)	172	37%

General supportive therapies
Treatment	N	% helped
Meditation/relaxation/prayer (18)	267	55%
Vitamin/mineral supplements (16)	290	48%
Herbal supplements (17)	217	39%
Homeopathy (13)	187	36%
Chiropractic manipulation (15)	181	33%
Acupuncture (14)	132	26%

Specific therapies
Treatment	N	% helped
Antifungal candida therapy (19)	234	41%
Avoid electromagnetic fields (21)	165	33%
Mercury amalgam removal (20)	112	28%
Parasite therapy (22)	82	28%
Coffee enemas (24)	47	28%
Colonics (23)	70	24%
Juicing (35)	75	23%
Ultra-Clear (41)	66	18%
Hydrogen peroxide therapy (43)	59	12%

Supplements
Treatment	N	% helped
Vitamin C: non-ester (29)	221	43%
Digestive enzymes (34)	212	35%
Vitamin C: ester (28)	161	34%
DHEA (38)	57	30%
Thyroid supplements (37)	147	30%
Acidophilus (33)	248	30%
Echinacea (36)	163	26%
Garlic (Kyolic) (31)	168	25%
Coenzyme Q10 (normal dose) (32)	137	21%
L-Glutathione (reduced) (39)	80	20%
Garlic (raw) (30)	158	17%
Sunrider herbal products (40)	46	7%
KM (42)	35	6%

Legend: ■ Enormous help ■ Major help

Continued next page

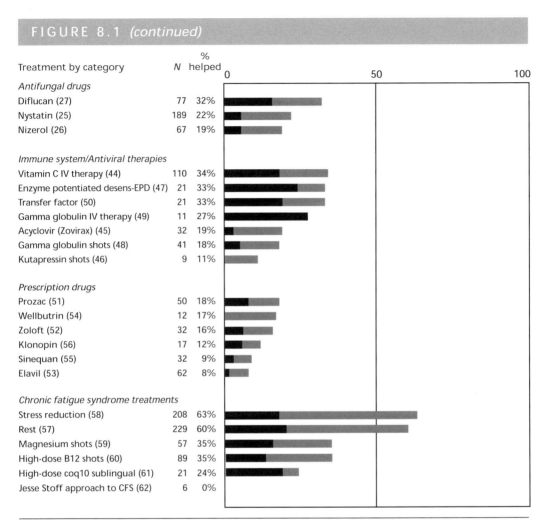

FIGURE 8.1 *(continued)*

Treatment by category	N	% helped
Antifungal drugs		
Diflucan (27)	77	32%
Nystatin (25)	189	22%
Nizerol (26)	67	19%
Immune system/Antiviral therapies		
Vitamin C IV therapy (44)	110	34%
Enzyme potentiated desens-EPD (47)	21	33%
Transfer factor (50)	21	33%
Gamma globulin IV therapy (49)	11	27%
Acyclovir (Zovirax) (45)	32	19%
Gamma globulin shots (48)	41	18%
Kutapressin shots (46)	9	11%
Prescription drugs		
Prozac (51)	50	18%
Wellbutrin (54)	12	17%
Zoloft (52)	32	16%
Klonopin (56)	17	12%
Sinequan (55)	32	9%
Elavil (53)	62	8%
Chronic fatigue syndrome treatments		
Stress reduction (58)	208	63%
Rest (57)	229	60%
Magnesium shots (59)	57	35%
High-dose B12 shots (60)	89	35%
High-dose coq10 sublingual (61)	21	24%
Jesse Stoff approach to CFS (62)	6	0%

Treatment efficacy rated by patients with multiple chemical sensitivities (MCS). Data derived from LeRoy, Haney Davis, & Jason (1996).

cancer (Kritchevsky, 1995). Furthermore, pharmaceutical companies are unlikely to fund research on alternative treatments, such as vitamin supplements, because they cannot claim proprietary rights over their manufacture and distribution, whereas vitamin supplement producers are not federally required to clinically test their products for efficacy.

In another study of patient-rated treatments, the research team at DePaul University recently completed a survey of treatments by 305 individuals with multiple chemical sensitivities (MCS), 41% of whom also had CFS (LeRoy, Haney Davis, & Jason, 1996). MCS is an illness reaction provoked by exposure to chemical and other irritants at levels well below those tolerated by individuals without this disorder. Individuals with MCS react to many of the products found in the average workplace and home. Their ratings of the most useful and least useful treatments are shown in Figure 8.1. In treatments specifically designed for people with MCS, 93% were helped by chemical sensitivity avoidance, and 86% were helped by creating environmentally safe homes. In a subsequent study by Davis, Jason, and Banghart (in press), individuals with MCS who lived in environmentally safe housing were significantly less disabled on two outcome measures.

The next treatment category in Figure 8.1 is Education, Support, and Growth. The highest priority areas were reading information about MCS (81%) and meeting other people with MCS (69%). In the next category, General Supportive Therapies, only meditation/relaxation/prayer was endorsed by more than 50% of the respondents. Because fewer than 50% of respondents endorsed the categories of Specific Therapies, Supplements, Anti-Fungal Drugs, Immune System/Anti-Viral Therapies, and Prescription Drugs, it is clear there is no single treatment approach that seems to work with the majority of MCS participants, except for the (nonmedical) avoidance strategies and meditation/relaxation/prayer, as mentioned earlier.

The last heading in Figure 8.1, Chronic Fatigue Syndrome Treatments, reveals that the two highest rated items were stress reduction (63%) and rest (60%). Many CFS patients mention that reducing stress and increasing rest are among the best strategies for reducing and controlling symptoms (Berne, 1992).

Conclusion

Given the multifaceted nature of CFS, it may be more productive to view the syndrome and its treatment within a biopsychosocial perspective. Perhaps promising biological therapies, such as Ampligen and dietary interventions, as indicated in Table 8.1, need to be combined with psychosocial interventions that focus on stress reduction and lifestyle adjustments in order to maximize positive clinical outcomes.

Cognitive-Behavioral Intervention 9

Once clinical assessment has confirmed a diagnosis of CFS and any concurrent psychological disorder, a therapeutic intervention may be designed that targets prominent stress symptoms and the underlying emotional issues. The published studies of psychological intervention in CFS have all used cognitive–behavioral approaches. Although the clinical procedures were different and the therapeutic outcomes inconsistent among these studies, important treatment suggestions can be derived from the data. This chapter begins with a critical review of the published clinical outcome studies in CFS (see Table 9.1). Then the proposed link between stress and fatigue in CFS is described as the conceptual basis for the cognitive and behavioral coping techniques that are subsequently presented in this chapter. These interventions include relaxation techniques, pleasant mood induction and maintenance, activity pacing, daily life restructuring and graded activity, cognitive coping, social support, and memory assistance.

Therapeutic Outcome Studies in CFS

An initial open trial (S. Butler et al., 1991) of cognitive–behavioral treatment for 27 moderately disabled CFS patients showed dramatic reductions in symptom severity

TABLE 9.1

Studies of Cognitive–Behavioral Intervention in CFS

Authors	Design	N	Number of sessions	Intervention	Clinical outcome
S. Butler et al., 1991	Single-group clinical trial	27	7–8	Graded activity	Significant improvements: Fatigue and functional status maintained at 3-month follow-up.
Lloyd et al., 1993	Randomized, double-blind placebo controlled trial	90	6	Graded activity, immunotherapy	No significant treatment effect. No follow-up.
Friedberg & Krupp, 1994	Multigroup clinical trial	64	6	Coping skills	Significant improvements: Depression symptoms and maladaptive illness beliefs. No follow-up.
Sharpe et al., 1996	Randomized controlled trial	60	16	Graded activity	Significant improvements: Fatigue and functional status at 6- and 12-month follow-up.
Deale et al., 1997	Randomized controlled trial	60	13	Graded activity	Significant improvements: Fatigue and functional status at 6-month follow-up.
Fulcher & White, 1997	Randomized controlled trial	66	12	Graded aerobic exercise	Significant improvements: fatigue, functional capacity and fitness. Greater improvements at 3- and 12-month follow-up.

and disability. One third of treated patients became symptom free during posttreatment. The outcome data were consistent with the authors' treatment assumptions that reversible psychological factors maintained CFS symptoms. The treatment approach focused on graded activity, that is, setting up behavioral schedules for patients beginning at a very low level of exertion and progressively increasing activity until therapeutic goals were achieved. For instance, a home-bound patient would presumably learn to increase activity gradually until he or she could take a walk or go shopping and perhaps resume working part-time. It was assumed that physical disability was maintained by a fear of symptom flare-ups associated with physical exertion and activity. Additionally, it was proposed that the lack of activity engendered a physically deconditioned state, leaving the patient more vulnerable to activity-induced symptom exacerbations.

The shortcomings of the S. Butler et al. (1991) study included a high dropout rate of 31%, a nonstandardized treatment duration, and the absence of a control group. It is also plausible that this clinical sample represented a subset of CFS patients who have significant fatigue attributable to psychobehavioral factors (Friedberg & Krupp, 1995). For instance, the S. Butler et al. (1991) sample was similar in therapeutic response to a clinically depressed group without CFS in a cognitive–behavioral treatment study (Friedberg & Krupp, 1994). Finally, 38% of the original patients were lost to follow-up (Bonner, Ron, Chalder, Butler, & Wessely, 1994), which further limits the generalizability of the findings (Lipkin et al., 1995).

In a subsequent study (Lloyd et al., 1993), cognitive–behavioral treatment of CFS was compared with immunological therapy in a double-blind placebo controlled trial ($N = 90$). On the POMS, no significant differences were found on the subscales of depression, anxiety, or fatigue severity between placebo, immunological therapy (dialyzable leucocyte, i.e., transfer factor) and cognitive–behavioral treatment. Also, no treatment effect was noted on measures of functional status or daily nonsedentary activity. The cognitive–behavioral intervention adopted the assumption of S. Butler et al., (1991) that psychological maintaining factors in CFS could be reversed with an active behavioral intervention, based on graduated activity schedules combined with desensitization of a phobic-like avoidance to CFS symptoms.

Due to the strong design of the Lloyd et al. (1993) study, further analysis is warranted. The treatment protocol described a structured stepwise behavioral intervention to mobilize patients. This graded activity formulation would be appropriate if activity were avoided due to depressed mood, an unrealistic fear of symptom flare-ups, or simple physical deconditioning. It is not clear from the Lloyd et al. (1993) study if psychological avoidance of activity was merely assumed or actually identified. However, for those individuals with CFS who do not have psychologically or behaviorally mediated reductions in activity, such a directed approach might be inappropriate and perhaps counterproductive.

The applicability of physical exercise to patients with CFS is also an unresolved issue. The behavioral intervention of physical exercise, aerobic or nonaerobic, has been shown to be an effective therapy for depression in numerous studies (Martinson, 1987). Clinically depressed individuals without CFS do not report an intolerance of exercise but rather have lost the desire to engage in activity generally

(American Psychiatric Association, 1994). In contrast, 79–87% of CFS individuals reported prolonged fatigue after exercise that would have been easily tolerated premorbidly (Friedberg et al., 1994; Komaroff et al., 1996). Although physical deconditioning from inactivity has been suggested as a partial explanation for activity avoidance in CFS (S. Butler et al., 1991; Fischler, Dendale, et al., 1997), a study of graded exercise testing in CFS compared with age and sex match controls found no evidence for physical deconditioning (Montague, Marie, Klassen, Bewick, & Horacek, 1989). In the absence of consistent empirical data, prescription of exercise must be based on sensitive clinical judgment, as we describe in the discussion that follows.

In a multigroup clinical study, Friedberg and Krupp (1994) compared results of a cognitive–behavioral coping skills intervention for patients with CFS and primary depression. The study consisted of three groups: a CFS treated group ($n = 22$), a primary depression treatment group ($n = 20$), and a no-treatment control group of participants with CFS ($n = 22$). The treatment was focused on identification of symptom relapse triggers, activity modification to minimize setbacks, acquisition of cognitive and behavioral coping skills, stress reduction and relaxation techniques, and group social support. Outcome data revealed a trend toward reduced depression scores and significant reductions in catastrophic thinking about fatigue in the CFS treatment group, but no significant reductions in self-reported stress symptoms or fatigue severity scores. In the depression group, highly significant reductions ($p < .0001$) in depression, stress, and fatigue severity scores were found. No significant changes in any measure were observed in the untreated CFS group.

When a median split of depression scores was analyzed in the CFS treated group, significant reductions in depression, stress, and fatigue severity were found in the more highly depressed subgroup of CFS participants. Although fatigue was significantly reduced in this subgroup, it still remained abnormally high compared with healthy individuals and depressed patients. These findings are important because they suggest that for CFS patients, relieving depression with cognitive–behavioral treatment does not cure fatigue symptoms.

The Friedberg and Krupp (1994) study design was limited by non-randomization of the treatment and no-treatment conditions and the absence of follow-up data. Also, Chalder, Deale, and Wessely (1995) have stated that the absence of a graded activity component in this study may have reduced the potential for clinical improvements in the CFS treated sample. Friedberg and Krupp (1995) replied that graded activity was rejected by treated patients who reported that they were exhausting themselves with daily activities and therefore could not tolerate a schedule of increasing activities.

Finally, two randomized controlled trials of graded activity in CFS (Deale et al., 1997; Sharpe et al., 1996) reported substantial improvements in functioning and fatigue symptoms. In the Sharpe et al. (1996) study, a 16-session cognitive–behavioral intervention ($N = 60$) was compared with routine medical care alone for CFS. Substantial improvements (Karnofsky performance rating; Karnofsky et al., 1948) in symptoms and disabilities were evidenced in 73% of the cognitive–behavioral treatment condition, but only 27% of the medical-care-only condition. The magnitude of improvement increased markedly over the 12-month follow-up period. An important cognitive component of the therapy encouraged attribution of the illness to psychosocial influences rather than organic factors. Clinical interventions also included gradual increases in activity, coping strategies to reduce perfectionism and self-criticism, and practical problem-solving techniques.

It is important to note that the cognitive–behavioral treatment group in the Sharpe et al. (1996) study were largely disabled from working (87%) and spent about half of their waking hours in bed. Given such high levels of functional impairment and the finding that anxiety and depression at intake were important predictors of outcome (Sharpe, 1996), it is possible that psychiatric morbidity rather than a CFS disease process maintained disability and symptom status. In addition, preliminary findings in psychological studies of CFS have found that higher levels of impairment have been associated with perceptions of helplessness (Ray et al., 1995a) that may be reinforced by significant others (Schmaling & DiClementi, 1995). These reversible psychosocial factors may be treated in CFS—although a near-complete resolution of the illness, as reported in Sharpe et al. (1996)—suggests the presence in many patients of primary psychiatric illness with prominent fatigue symptoms, rather than CFS.

In the third controlled, randomized cognitive–behavioral treatment study of CFS ($N = 60$; Deale et al., 1997), graded activity was compared with relaxation techniques over a 13-session treatment period. Daily activity schedules were assigned and completed by the graded activity group, regardless of symptom interference. For instance, one severely disabled patient was told to sit up in bed and eat supper with the family every day (Wessely, 1996). Fifty-three percent of the graded activity group were rated "much improved" and 20% "improved" in physical functioning, compared with19% of those in the relaxation group. As in the Sharpe et al. (1996) study, the greatest improvements occurred during the 12-month follow-up interval. It should be noted that the first three sessions in the cognitive–behavioral intervention involved engaging the patients in therapy rather than implementing an aggressive treatment plan. Then, the initial intervention was formulated, which in some cases involved *reducing* activity. Only after a schedule of consistent rest and activity was established were levels of activity increased. These initial steps in therapy to engage the patient over several visits and then redistribute or reduce activity were not emphasized in the published report. It suggests that the graded activity method was replaced for some patients with the more flexible approach of activity pacing, a coping skills technique used in a previously cited study (Friedberg & Krupp, 1994).

Based on these latter two graded activity studies, a recent prestigious report from the Royal College of Physicians, Psychiatrists and General Practitioners in Great Britain (Report of a Joint Working Group, 1996) stated that "the controlled increases in activity remain the cornerstone of the management of CFS" (p. 24) and that "rest per se is contraindicated in CFS" (p. 26).

Finally, a randomized controlled trial of graded exercise in 66 patients with CFS (Fulcher & White, 1997) showed significant improvements in fatigue, functional capacity, and physical fitness in a majority of patients. The percentage of patients rating themselves as better increased at 3- and 12-month follow-up evaluations. Seventy-five percent of patients returned to premorbid activity levels. It should be noted that 20 patients were taking full dosage antidepressants throughout the trial. As CFS patients have been observed to be quite sensitive to medications (Francis, 1990) and often report adverse reactions to even subclinical dosages (Twemlow et al., 1997), it is surprising that these participants could tolerate standard clinical regimens of antidepressants. The differential diagnosis of CFS and psychiatric disorder is difficult to judge in this study, and the possibility of primary undiagnosed psychiatric disorder remains a possibility.

Explaining Clinical Outcomes

How can the divergence in the aforementioned clinical findings be explained? A plausible reason why one of the graded activity studies (Lloyd et al., 1993) and the coping skills intervention (Friedberg & Krupp, 1994) did not yield more substantial outcomes is that the treatment duration in both studies was only six sessions, and no follow-up assessments were done. By contrast, the successful graded activity and exercise studies involved 8–16 sessions. Also, clinical outcomes in the controlled studies (Deale et al., 1997; Fulcher & White, 1997; Sharpe et al., 1996) were most significant at follow-up assessments, not at treatment termination.

The heterogeneity of the CFS population may be another factor that is related to clinical outcome. In the three successful graded activity reports (S. Butler et al., 1991; Deale et al., 1997; Sharpe et al., 1996), patients were moderately to severely disabled (most were unemployed; many were bedridden) and showed a high frequency of psychiatric morbidity. In contrast, participants in the coping skills study (Friedberg & Krupp, 1994) were relatively high-functioning (most were employed) and less disabled by psychiatric disorders, even though the majority of these participants evidenced psychiatric disorders. Some severely debilitated patients may respond favorably to graded activity because they are more likely to be disabled by psychiatric symptoms such as anxiety and depression (Hickie et al., 1995) that are reversible with behavioral interventions. In contrast, high-functioning CFS patients who maintain employment and other activities have already achieved many of the goals of graded activity and therefore may be more appropriately treated with coping skills for intrusive symptoms and limitations. A direct comparison of graded activity and coping skills interventions for high- and low-functioning CFS patients would be necessary to confirm the validity of this subgrouping hypothesis.

Cognitive–Behavioral Intervention in the Clinical Setting

CFS patients will often resist seeing a mental health professional because they believe that it erroneously validates a psychological explanation of their illness. Initially, the behavioral clinician may hear these patients express the anger they feel toward physicians and others who have classified their complaints as a psychological or quasi-psychological disorder (C. Butler & Rollnick, 1996). Such disbelief on the part of others is a major source of stress that for many patients is as damaging as the illness itself (McKenzie et al., 1995):

> Being disbelieved and ignored, it's more difficult to deal with than the illness itself. The word has got to get out to employers and the public that there are illnesses that are disabling but don't have that appearance.

> The hardest thing has been the laughter at our expense, having to pretend to others, to not even tell on a doctor's form that I have CFS for fear that he will dismiss me as a depressed person

It's so frustrating to feel like death warmed over but to look good. (Friedberg, 1995c, p. 87)

What is most important to patients initially is an unequivocal empathic response from the treating clinician to their complaints. CFS-affected individuals want a sense of illness validation and support after numerous experiences of rejection and dismissal by physicians and others (C. Butler & Rollnick, 1996).

In this section, a stress–fatigue model serves as the conceptual basis for a coping skills–oriented cognitive–behavioral intervention in CFS. This type of intervention can reduce depression, anxiety, and—to a lesser extent—fatigue in CFS, as well as improve coping abilities. It is not as clear that coping skills treatment can improve daily functioning, although behavioral techniques can reduce the frequency and severity of relapses. As argued earlier, the England-based reports of functional improvements in CFS using graded activity may be valid for a subset of CFS patients who are characterized by high levels of disability and psychiatry morbidity. This subgroup may represent a significant minority of CFS patients (cf. Hickie et al., 1995). Our impression is that most individuals with CFS are usually doing as much as they can, given the limitations imposed by the illness. A wide range of disability is found in CFS from bedridden confinement to limitation in one domain only, such as physical exercise or neuro-cognitive functioning. It is important to assess what the patient can and cannot do so as to fully understand the restrictions of the illness. Thus, the patient should be queried about limitations in vocational, family, social, recreational, and exercise activities.

The Stress–Fatigue Link in CFS

Since fatigue, similar to pain, is a symptom that may be strongly influenced by psychological factors, our clinical interventions for CFS are modeled after cognitive–behavioral treatment of chronic pain (Turk, Meichenbaum, & Genest, 1983). Cognitive–behavioral therapy of chronic fatigue is based on the assumption that fatigue-related thoughts and behaviors are operants that can be constructively altered with cognitive reevaluation and behavioral prescription. Figure 9.1 illustrates the behavioral, cognitive, and emotional sequence of stress creation in CFS.

The patient with CFS can be seen as having sustained a major reduction in positive reinforcement. The range of activities that had previously produced positive effects is instead accompanied or

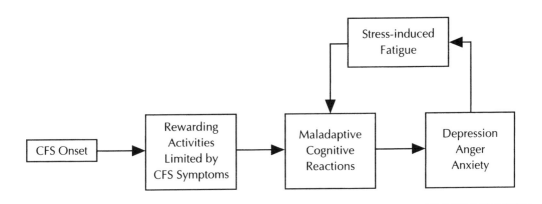

Model of affective distress in CFS.

followed by fatigue (Fordyce, 1976). Fatigue and its associated disability trigger illness-related cognitive distortions such as exaggerated catastrophic beliefs, self-deprecation, and intolerance of symptoms (Ellis, 1962, 1997; Ellis & Abrams, 1994). These understandable, if maladaptive, beliefs elicit negative emotions such as depression or discouragement, anger, and anxiety (Ellis, 1962). Additional fatigue is associated with these emotions (American Psychiatric Association, 1994). Therefore, by restricting the range of activities to avoid severe fatigue and then reacting to symptoms and limitations with stress-producing thoughts, the patient establishes a cycle of emotional stress,

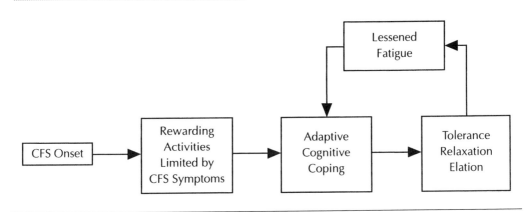

Model of healthy coping in CFS.

more fatigue, and sustained emotional stress (see Figure 9.1; Friedberg, 1995d). In a recent qualitative study of 66 CFS patients (Clements, Sharpe, Simkin, Borrill, & Hawton, 1997), the majority of patients believed that "stress" played a role in their illness.

As conceptualized for CFS, coping skills–focused cognitive–behavioral therapy restructures the linkage between illness-related disability and its consequences of maladaptive cognitions and fatigue-related affect. Fatigue-induced emotional stress and depression are treated with relaxation techniques and pleasant mood induction; maladaptive cognitions with cognitive coping skills and interpersonal support; and symptom fluctuations and disability with activity pacing, daily life structuring, and social assertiveness training. A model of healthy coping with CFS is presented in Figure 9.2. Clearly, the interventions prescribed will vary with the emotional and functional status of the individual patient. A structured eight-session protocol for coping skills treatment of CFS groups is described in chapter 11.

It is important to inform clients that any emotional or physical stress, even a relatively minor one, may substantially increase their fatigue (Wood et al., 1994). Typically, a series of minor stressors will cumulatively increase fatigue and stress symptoms. Clients can control stress and its effect on CFS symptoms with cognitive and behavioral techniques that counteract stress and help to restore emotional well-being. First, it is important that the client identify stress–fatigue connections. A daily stress log kept for one week will sharpen the patient's recognition of specific stressors and how they affect mood and symptoms (see Table 7.1).

The standard coping techniques described in the discussion that follows are specifically focused on CFS treatment. As defined for CFS, effective coping is a process of behavioral adaptation to a stressor that is associated with reductions in distress, increased tolerance of the stressor, a greater sense of well-being, and a heightened feeling of self-control (Friedberg, 1995b; see Figure 9.2). An impressive number of studies show that a personal sense of control or mastery both (a) directly reduces psychological disturbance and the symptoms of physical illness and (b) buffers the deleterious effects of stress exposure on physical and mental health (Thoits, 1995).

Relaxation Training

For the CFS patient, relaxation is an important ameliorative agent (Friedberg, 1995c) for the chronic stress, tension, and anxiety often associated with the illness (Friedberg & Krupp, 1994; McKenzie et al., 1995).

Calming techniques also create a sense of well-being for the chronically ill, a finding recently confirmed in CFS patients (Friedberg & Krupp, 1994). Relaxation training in healthy individuals has been associated with selected improvements in immune function (Kiecolt-Glaser & Glaser, 1992), an important point for CFS sufferers because immunological defects associated with CFS (Klonoff, 1992) may be a contributing cause of the illness.

Clients may be instructed to use relaxation as a coping skill for daily stress in relation to family, work, and social involvements as well as to illness-related stressors. To facilitate effective relaxation, clients are told to become aware of the early signs of stressful feelings such as mild headache, stiffness in the neck, nervous or tight feelings in the stomach, jittery sensations, and restlessness. A relaxation technique may diffuse these initial sensations before stress symptoms become intense and less manageable. As a sleep induction technique, relaxation can hasten sleep onset and reduce nighttime awakenings that compromise a full night's sleep. Prescribed relaxation may also facilitate reevaluation of unhealthy self-demands to overdo activity that may be associated with setbacks or relapses. Finally, focused relaxation can reduce mental confusion and restore greater clarity to the patient's thinking processes (Friedberg, 1995c).

CFS patients often resist taking the time to practice home relaxation because they think it is a waste of time (Friedberg, 1995c). Quiet time might be viewed as an unnecessary indulgence that is incompatible with active completion of tasks. A lingering sense of guilt about activity restrictions also deters relaxation time. Client opposition to self-focused leisure is consistent with personality data in CFS studies suggesting the presence of compulsive traits (Pepper et al., 1993), a personality characteristic of "action proneness" (Van Houdenhove et al., 1995), "hard-driving" tendencies (Lewis, Cooper, & Bennett, 1994) and overcommitted lifestyles (N. C. Ware, 1993). Cognitive coping statements that will promote a more constructive attitude about relaxation include "I am entitled to take time for myself"; "Relaxation will improve my mood and my coping ability"; "Relaxation benefits me and those around me—that makes sense"; "Relaxation will make me more efficient."

The following personal account from a 34-year-old female CFS patient with two children illustrates the difficulty in taking time for relaxation:

> I learned the relaxation technique in therapy, which was OK, but practicing it at home was a pain at first. There are so many other things I have to do! But by doing the relaxation I began to realize how stressed I was getting just doing all my housework and taking care of the kids when they got home. The relaxation helped me get off the daily "treadmill." It eased some of the mental and

physical exhaustion. I also felt less irritable and snappy with the kids, which has been a big problem since I got sick.

BREATHING FOCUS

A straightforward relaxation technique that is easily learned by the patient is "breathing focus." Sitting in a comfortable chair, such as a recliner, the client thinks the syllables *re* during the inhale and *lax* during the exhale. This exercise should be done in a comfortable, quiet setting with minimal distractions. The *relax* phrase should be practiced for two 10-minute periods a day, once in the morning and once in the afternoon, before meals. Usually within a few days the patient will begin to feel the release of tension and stress and experience feelings of calm and well-being.

A relaxation script that includes the breathing focus follows. It may be used in session and taped for the client to use at home:

> One, let your eyes close. Two, take a long, deep breath, and three, slowly release the breath. Feel the release, the letting go as you exhale and allow your breathing to assume an easy, natural rhythm. Focus on the easy breathing rhythm . . . inhale and exhale. Simply observe it and recognize it as a natural process, an easy response and a source of relaxation. . . . Observation is simply passive attention to your own natural rhythms. Appreciate them. . . . Now focus on the release of breath. Each time you exhale, you release tension as well as breathe. With each exhale, there is a perceptible release of tension, as well as breath. Exhale, release; exhale, release. . . . Feel the release, the letting go that accompanies each release of breath. Exhale, release. . . . Now allowing relaxed feelings to radiate upward . . . to the shoulders, going across the shoulders and descending through both arms. Upper arms relaxed . . . lower arms relaxed . . . both arms relaxing. Now relaxed feelings descending through the chest, flowing into the stomach, the stomach becoming relaxed. Relaxed sensations spreading through the hips and to the upper legs and enveloping the upper legs. Now flowing to the lower legs . . . all the way down to the feet. The feet becoming loose and relaxed, loose and relaxed. Relaxed sensations retracing their gentle path upward. Lower legs relaxed . . . upper legs relaxed. Relaxed feelings ascending the lower back, lower back loosening . . . Now proceeding to the upper back . . . up the back of the neck . . . infusing the area with relaxed sensations. Now spreading up over the scalp and down the face . . . forehead relaxed, eyes relaxed, jaw becoming loose, limp, and slack; loose, limp, and slack.
>
> You have reached a pleasant plateau of calm and comfort. Recognize the feelings you now have. Know that you can reproduce these feelings with regular easy practice. . . .
>
> Now, as I count from 1 to 10, you can feel even more relaxed: 1, more relaxed; 2, even more; 3, deeper down; 4, more

relaxed; 5, calmer still; 6, even more; 7, deeper down; 8, more relaxed; 9, so very calm; 10, your entire physical self completely immersed in relaxed sensations . . . calm, wavy deep relaxation, so deeply and comfortably relaxed.[1]

Now refocus on the easy breathing rhythm, the source of profound release and relaxation. As you inhale, say to yourself, *reee*. . . . And as you exhale, *laaax*. . . . A long *reee* as you inhale and a slow *laax* as you exhale. *Ree Laax.* Now I'd like you to take the next minute to say the *re-lax* phrase to yourself along with your breathing. Go ahead now and my voice will return shortly. (Pause for one minute)

All right. Very good. Continue relaxing and recognize the feelings you now have at this deeper level. Recognize your ability to reproduce these feelings with regular easy practice.

Now, when it is comfortable for you, slowly open your eyes, bringing yourself back to wakefulness; Feeling relaxed and refreshed.

PLEASANT IMAGERY

Some clients prefer a relaxation technique that focuses on pleasant imagery such as the beach, the country, or the mountains (Golden, Gersch, & Robbins, 1991; Siegel, 1986). Such visualizations may be more effective for clients who experience "racing" thoughts and an inability to directly relax their thinking with body-focused techniques such as breathing focus. These clients may respond better to the distraction provided by imagined pleasant scenes. Although these techniques may be as effective as breathing focus, the breathing method has the advantage of "portability." It can be used quickly and easily as a coping skill in many situations.

If the patient has difficulty relaxing with breathing focus, or would like to enhance their relaxation experience, the following transcript of a beach scene can also be incorporated into the therapy session or recorded as a taped exercise:

Imagine yourself spending an afternoon at the beach. The sand feels warm and soft against your skin. You are sitting on the sand observing the ocean, the azure blue water, viewing the flow of the waves as they move rhythmically to the shore, the water becoming a light transparent green as it flows to the shoreline. And you see the whitecaps on the waves as the waves roll onto the shore; yes, waves gently reaching the shore, like sparkling water spilling on the sand; feeling a salty, refreshing spray in the

---

[1]From *Coping With Chronic Fatigue Syndrome: Nine Things You Can Do* (pp. 67–68), by F. Friedberg, 1995, Oakland, CA: New Harbinger. Copyright 1995 by New Harbinger Publications. Reprinted with permission.

air, that refreshing misty spray permeating your body—so wonderfully invigorating and uplifting, revitalizing and relaxing.

Allow yourself the next few moments to imagine the pleasant flow of the waves onto the shore as they rise and fall, rise and fall. Go ahead now and imagine the waves.
(Pause for about 5 seconds.)

All right. Very good. Now you decide to take an easy stroll along the beach as you view the surf; yes, observe the curving shoreline off in the distance, the curving shoreline as it merges with the horizon. As you walk onward, onward, you feel the sand crunching beneath your feet; such a pleasant sensation—the warm, crunchy sand. It complements the warmth of the sun overhead. Feel the warmth of the sun on your back, that gentle warmth flowing down your back and throughout your body; comfortable warmth from the sun filling you with pleasant sensations. With your senses so very aware, you notice the sand dunes rising along the beach, sand dunes with isolated clumps of tall grass on their slopes. Noticing the tall grass gently swaying in the breeze. The breezes creating tranquil feelings.

And as you walk onward, you hear the sound of seagulls in the distance. A flock of white seagulls approaching, flying so easily, gliding in the wind, making their distinctive sounds passing overhead. Now flying off in the distance, leaving you with a feeling of serenity. . . . Now feeling a gentle breeze at your back. The gentle breeze coaxing you further along, heightening your senses.

As you look across the waves, you see a sleek white sailboat moving through the water. The boat moving so gracefully, the sails filled with gently sweeping winds. Enjoy the silent steadiness of the boat as it moves along with the wind.

Now as you gaze further toward the horizon, you see the sun setting. Yes, the sun setting in a full display of vivid colors: bright yellows, deep reds, and burnt oranges against the light gray clouds and a pale blue sky. As the sun descends, it projects a long wedge of yellow light across the water; slowly sinking down. And a breathtaking serenity begins to pervade the atmosphere. An emerging serenity so deep that it is fully absorbing your senses.

Now you begin to conclude the experience—finish the experience with acceptance and peace, acceptance and peace. . . . Allow yourself the next minute, all the time in the world, all the time you need to bring yourself back to wakefulness, your eyes opening slowly, feeling relaxed and refreshed.[2]

HEALING IMAGERY

Despite the extensive media coverage on mind–body cures, there is no convincing evidence that relaxation or healing imagery will cure CFS

---

[2]From *Coping With Chronic Fatigue Syndrome: Nine Things You Can Do* (pp. 58–59), by F. Friedberg, 1995, Oakland, CA: New Harbinger. Copyright 1995 by New Harbinger Publications. Reprinted with permission.

or other chronic illnesses such as cancer or heart disease. However, some clients feel that healing imagery is a constructive way to "fight" the illness and generate hope. Thus, it can be a useful alternative or addition to standard relaxation techniques. The following transcript incorporates healing suggestions:

> Your healing can now begin, yes, your healing begins from within yourself. An inner radiance that begins as a mere speck of light, yes, an inner point of light and warmth . . . radiating strength and power . . . yes, the strength and power that grows warm and radiant . . . inner strength. Feel it, experience it fully, thoroughly, inner radiance growing stronger. . . . Ready now, yes ready to direct its healing strength towards your weakened system. Yes, the inner radiance directing its strength towards your body. Feel that inner sense of strength beginning, working within your body. Feeling revitalized, re-energized . . . strengthening as your inner radiance strengthens and energizes. Feel the warm, intense energy doing its work; reactivating, restoring your body . . . yes, restoring your body. Experience that strengthening fully, thoroughly, that inner boosting, growing even stronger now, stronger, more powerful than before. And as you feel that strength, you believe in yourself and your ability to succeed in your goal of rebuilding your body. Yes, believing in the strength of your thoughts, images, and the totality of your internal powers. You believe so strongly, feeling that boost even now, yes, yet remaining tolerant, letting time pass, knowing that any worthwhile goal takes time, any worthwhile goal. And you have resolved to accomplish your goal, believing you can . . . re-energizing, boosting your system. You hold firmly to that belief; yes, so firmly . . . feeling less fatigued . . . and this message remains with you, far beyond these words, far beyond these words. Now, slowly bringing yourself back to wakefulness, eyes opening gradually, feeling relaxed and refreshed.[3]

Pleasant Mood Induction as a Treatment Intervention

Pleasant mood induction involves imagining or participating in an activity that, based on prior experience, will uplift mood and create a pleasant or euphoric emotional state. In research on healthy adults, pleasant mood induction has produced elation and healthy changes in stress hormones, as well as feelings of increased energy or vigor, reduced anger, and improved pain tolerance (Brown, 1993).

---

[3]From *Coping With Chronic Fatigue Syndrome: Nine Things You Can Do* (pp. 70–71), by F. Friedberg, 1995, Oakland, CA: New Harbinger. Copyright 1995 by New Harbinger Publications. Reprinted with permission.

These findings have been partially replicated in CFS patients. In a 1-year prospective study of positive and negative life events assessed for 130 participants with CFS , the frequency of positive events was found to be associated with lower scores for fatigue, impairment, anxiety, and depression, while negative life events were associated with higher anxiety but were unrelated to other measures (Ray et al., 1995b). It was concluded that positive life events and experiences may contribute to the process of recovery in CFS, although their occurrence may also be facilitated by a prior reduction of symptom severity. In a related finding, optimism in CFS patients has been associated with resistance to relapse in a prospective study of the effects of a hurricane on CFS patients (Lutgendorf, Antoni, et al., 1995). These emotional benefits of a pleasant or optimistic mood can diffuse the persistent stress of CFS and may improve functioning at least temporarily. One CFS patient offered this example of pleasant mood induction:

> When I'm able to get into something, like CFS political activism, the symptoms move into the background. I don't notice them so much, and I just feel positive, uplifted. So if I get mentally involved with something in a positive way, I'll feel better for awhile. I may or may not crash later from the effort. But I would say it's worth the risk.

Our clinical experience is consistent with the preceding data: Generating a positive mood will allow the client to (a) divert attention from symptoms, (b) replace negative feelings with positive ones, (c) lessen fatigue symptoms, (d) minimize symptom magnification, and (e) improve functioning for several hours or perhaps several days. In effect, mood elevation will interrupt the fatigue–stress cycle that engenders fatigue and emotional stress (see Figure 9.1). For instance, in CFS stress management groups conducted by one of the authors (Friedberg), a sense of shared coping and camaraderie was evident during the initial session. In the second session, the group participants often reported reduced symptoms and substantially uplifted mood. It appeared that the group interaction had a powerful mood-elevating effect. For many of these patients, the group interaction was their first experience communicating with others who understood their illness. Also, the group agenda was organized so that illness complaints were accepted without judgment. In this context, constructive suggestions and behavioral assignments could be offered with support and reassurance.

Generating pleasant experiences and sustaining a positive mood may be more difficult for the chronically ill. Therefore, the patient may need guidance and support to activate mood improvements. We ask patients to make a list of low-effort, uplifting activities, such as listening to a captivating speaker, sharing an intimate moment with a spouse or close friend, taking a bath, sitting in the park, watching ducks on a pond, reading an absorbing story, and so forth. Clients then select 5 to 10 of the items from the list and schedule them for the coming week. This exercise may be an important first step toward restoring pleasurable experiences for both the severely disabled client with limited choices as well as for the high-functioning individual with CFS who simply does not allow time for leisurely enjoyment.

We also suggest, as an assignment, that clients compose a list of 10 things that make them laugh as another vehicle to create a pleasant mood. The therapist explains to clients that humor and laughter are powerful distractions from the stress of CFS and that laughter stimulates the production of endorphins, the body's natural painkillers. Furthermore, research on laughter (Berk, 1989; Klein, 1989) has shown that it can enhance immune function; counteract depression; and even substitute, to some extent, for aerobic exercise. Laughter is also a natural tension-reducer. It produces relaxation for up to 45 minutes afterward (Klein, 1989). With humor and laughter, patients can confront personal problems in a more relaxed and creative state of mind and body.

Sustaining a Pleasant, Energetic Mood

For the individual with CFS, a good mood may easily be disrupted by the stress of fluctuating symptoms; the burden of attempting to sustain daily activities; and the marital, financial, and vocational strains that often accompany the illness. It is important to advise patients that good moods can be prolonged if they learn to recognize and alter mood-breaking behaviors. In the following example, a 35-year-old woman with CFS describes how she recognized and halted a declining mood:

> My mood was really up after my daughter's dance recital and my husband's announcement that we could actually afford to take a nice vacation. The next day I started doing a variety of routine household chores, sprinting from one task to another and answering several phone calls. And I could feel my good mood succumbing to increased fatigue and malaise, those feelings that I think only people with CFS can really understand. When I realized this, I stopped myself and thought, "Do I really have to work at this speed? I don't have any great time pressure and I'm losing my precious good mood." So, I sat in the recliner and did my relaxation technique and then paced myself so that I didn't rush through things. And I recovered that good mood! It just took a change of course to get it back.

The following suggestions to clients are designed to interrupt the process of mood deterioration and restore pleasant affect (Friedberg, 1995c):

1. Watch for the early signs of mood lowering and the reasons behind it: a shift to negative thinking, a change in behavior to activities or responsibilities that are burdensome or an unpleasant interaction with other people.
2. At the earliest opportunity, choose to shift away from the mood-breaking activity.
3. To redirect your attention in a positive way, begin with a relaxation technique (see pp. 142–145) or simply take a breather in a way that is pleasing to you. This may require only a minute or two.
4. If you return to the original activity that compromised your mood, do it differently, perhaps more slowly, perhaps with more patience. Alternatively, you might want to reschedule it for another time when energy and mood are more resilient.

Activity Pacing

Activity pacing involves moderating activity to minimize (a) the typical pattern of overwork when energy levels are higher and (b) the postexertion behavioral collapse with its consequences of more stress, discouragement, and frustration. Although CFS patients are forced to reduce activity from premorbid levels, they may retain the same high standards of performance and use whatever energy they have to sustain the highest possible functioning. Higher levels of physical and mental energy may be quickly depleted with more active task completion to "make up" for prior periods of inactivity. The resulting exhaustion and collapse may require several hours to several days of substantially reduced activity levels plus bedrest. The pacing concept is based on the envelope theory (see pp. 150–158), which views perceived energy (the energy one has at any moment) and expended activity (the energy used up) as the important subjective states in CFS that need to be matched or balanced in order to maintain functioning and reduce the frequency of relapses.

In practical terms, pacing suggestions encourage the patient to set up a daily routine of short-term, flexible and attainable goals. Daily behavioral goals allow the individual with CFS to preserve a fragile self-esteem that is threatened by ongoing disability. Long-term plans may be retained to sustain hope, but they are not the primary focus of therapy. To reduce the frequency of setbacks and maintain energy, a useful pacing strategy involves scheduling rest intervals or relaxing diversions rather than working to exhaustion. In addition, patients are encouraged to be selective about activities in order to preserve energy. For example, patients may complain that social events such as parties or having houseguests trigger mental fatigue and cognitive confusion due to the stress of prolonged conversations with others. Limiting social obligations may require new assertive skills that can be taught by the treating professional.

Clinicians are advised to assess the client's receptivity to pacing suggestions and then develop specific behavioral prescriptions. The goal of pacing is to engender a balance between activity, rest, and leisure time in order to reduce the frequency and severity of relapses. In a questionnaire study of patients with scleroderma, a serious, progressive chronic disease (Westbrook, Gething, & Bradbury, 1987), patients who perceived themselves as having the ability to control relapses were more likely to have experienced remission of symptoms in the previous year. One person with CFS described her pacing schedule as follows:

> I've learned to moderate my enjoyments. Now I don't go out and work hard for five to six hours at a stretch. I work for two or three hours, and to me that's better, because I don't have to take a week off to recover. (Friedberg, 1995c, p. 76)

If the patient is able to do modest physical exercise such as walking or low-level weight lifting (2–10 lb.) without precipitating a setback, then a flexible regimen of exercise can be designed. Because prolonged fatigue after exercise is common in CFS, patients need to modify their exercise routine in order to minimize symptom flare-ups and reduced functioning. In patients with CFS who are able to work full-time, it may not be economically feasible to reduce working hours as a restorative pacing technique. In such cases, stress reduction and relaxation techniques, as described earlier, may be the most practical intervention to cope with the burden of obligatory work schedules.

Graded Activity and Daily Life Structuring

The intervention of graded activity may be most appropriate for severely disabled patients with comorbid depression or anxiety disorders. Successful graded activity interventions have been reported for moderately to severely disabled individuals who usually had concurrent psychiatric disorders (e.g., Sharpe et al., 1996). For these patients, a daily routine of low-level activity may help to counteract the disabling effects of depression, anxiety, and excessive sedentary behavior. Suggestions for daily life structuring might include changing from pajamas to daytime clothing, making breakfast, reading for a few minutes, and light housework. These low effort activities may lessen feelings of depression and increase a sense of mastery and self-control. A severely disabled CFS patient explained how she benefited from establishing a daily routine:

> When I first became ill, I was bedbound for days at a time, and my sleep was so disturbed that no amount of it seemed to restore any energy. And feelings of depression seemed to merge with my fatigue so I just felt this oppressive physical and emotional burden. But as I began to schedule my day by clearly differentiating night and sleeptime from day and simple activities, I started to be less dependent on others helping me. The progress has been slow, taking many months. However, it has allowed me to maintain some degree of steadiness in my energy levels, to regain some autonomy, and to do some of the activities that were formerly impossible.

A schedule of activities involving step-wise increments in physical exertion over several months may be attempted for very debilitated patients. Given the positive outcomes of the English-based graded activity studies (Deale et al., 1997; Sharpe et al., 1996), this type of intervention may hold promise for quality of life improvements. Our reluctance to endorse graded activity arises from our vastly different clinical experience with CFS patients in the United States. A replication of graded activity outcomes in a well-designed U.S. study would be necessary before we would recommend its general use in CFS populations.

Envelope Theory: Resolving the Rest–Activity Dilemma

Much of the controversy surrounding illness management in CFS reflects medical uncertainty over the appropriate balance between rest and activity. The concepts of energy conservation and activity moderation (Berne, 1992; Collinge, 1993; Swan, 1996) have emerged from this debate. It has been hypothesized that, if people with CFS are to begin the slow process of recovery, they must contain their levels of expended energy. Informally known as the "fifty-percent solution" (Collinge, 1993) or the "envelope theory," this hypothesis holds that, by keeping expended energy levels within the envelope of perceived energy levels, people with CFS can prevent relapse and possibly increase their energy levels. In other words, by not overexerting themselves, people with CFS can avoid exertion-related setbacks and relapses and, over time, increase their energy and tolerance of activity as well.

This model is timely, given the medical disagreement over the appropriate level of activity for patients with CFS. Rather than prescribing increased rest or activity universally to all patients with CFS, the envelope theory falls in the middle of the rest–activity debate. Under this model, the unique condition of each CFS patient is assessed. Suggestions for treatment plans and illness management are based upon these individualized assessments. For example, under the envelope theory, patients with CFS that continually overexert themselves would be advised to cut back and conserve their energy resources in order to achieve long-term gains in their tolerance to activity. On the other hand, people with CFS who are severely disabled and inactive for prolonged periods might be encouraged to gradually increase activity as tolerance develops. Thus envelope theory promotes the use of moderation and energy conservation based on individualized treatment programs.

A CASE STUDY OF ENVELOPE THEORY

A case report by King, Jason, Frankenberry, Jordan, and Tryon (1997) was conducted to empirically test the principles of the envelope theory and to explore the relationships between perceived levels of energy, expended levels of energy, and fatigue. This CFS case illustrates how fluctuations in fatigue are related to activity and energy levels and to affective states. These interrelationships are then examined to identify illness management strategies.

For a 16-month period, beginning in the spring of 1995, data were collected on a daily basis for one individual with CFS. Each day, the CFS participant was asked to rate levels of fatigue on a 100-point scale (0 = *no fatigue*, 100 = *extreme fatigue*), perceived energy (0 = *no energy*, 100 = *abundant energy*, similar to his condition when he was completely well), and expended energy (0 = *no energy expended or used up*, 100 = *all energy expended or used up*). In addition to the daily ratings made by the participant, hourly ratings of the symptoms and activities were made from 6 a.m. to 8 p.m. for several days during initial data collection. During these several days, the participant was asked to follow the energy-conserving strategy of maintaining his perceived and expended energy at roughly the same levels. Feedback based on the figures below was used to help guide this behavior change intiative.

In an effort to reduce the large amount of hourly data collected,

FIGURE 9.3

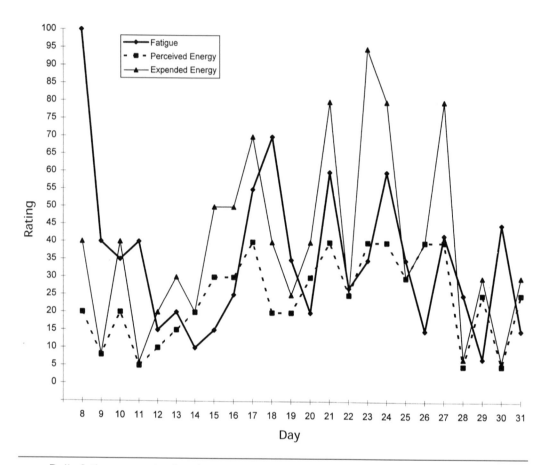

Daily fatigue, perceived and expended energy for spring of 1995.

we selected particular days of the hourly data to illustrate our major findings. The first visual analysis, presented in Figure 9.3, shows the covarying relationship between fatigue, perceived energy, and expended energy for the first month of data collection. During this month, levels of expended energy ($M = 39\%$) tended to greatly exceed levels of perceived energy ($M = 24\%$). As a result, the degree of fatigue ($M = 35\%$) experienced by the participant remained consistently high despite periodic fluctuations. This first month of data represents an example of energy overexertion and the consequent high levels of fatigue.

This relationship between perceived energy, expended energy, and fatigue can be seen more clearly on a hourly basis. Shown in Figure 9.4 are hourly ratings for fatigue, perceived energy, and expended

FIGURE 9.4

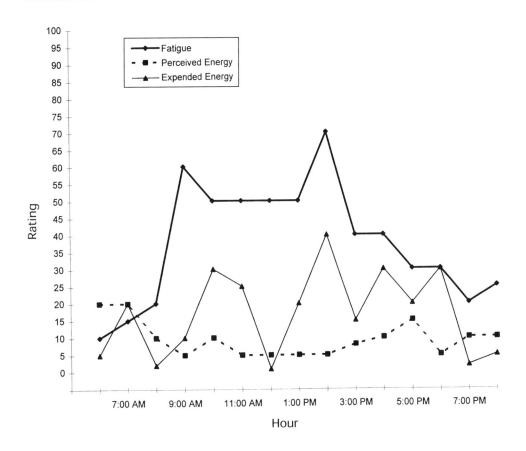

Hourly fatigue, perceived and expended energy for spring of 1995.

energy for one day. On this day, the participant's levels of expended energy were higher than his levels of perceived energy on 9 out of 15 hourly ratings. Given this degree of overexertion, fatigue levels were elevated throughout the day, ranging from moderate to high. (It is interesting that the hourly ratings for fatigue, negative affect, and positive affect were unrelated. Thus, affective states for the participant do not appear to influence levels of fatigue [see Figure 9.5].)

In Figure 9.4, it appears that the desired low levels of fatigue in the beginning of the day did not last, because the participant expended more energy than was optimal. By comparison, fatigue also began at a relatively low level as shown in Figure 9.6, but it stayed at a low level because the participant's expended energy remained safely below his perceived energy for the entire morning. In other words, the partici-

FIGURE 9.5

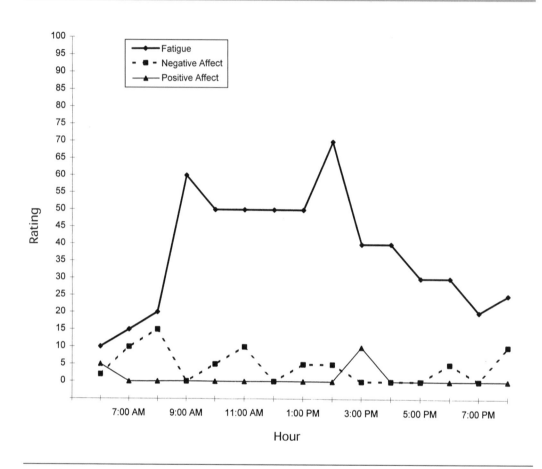

Hourly fatigue, negative and positive affect for spring of 1995.

pant, by not overexerting himself, conserved energy. However, once expended energy began to exceed perceived energy (approximately 1:00 p.m.; see Figure 9.6), fatigue rose sharply from a rating of 15 at 1:00 p.m. to a rating of 40 at 5:00 p.m. Then, the individual initiated a coping response: Shortly after 5:00 p.m., he reduced expended energy below the level of perceived energy. This coping behavior reduced energy overexpenditures and was successful in alleviating fatigue during the evening hours (see Figure 9.6).

Figure 9.7 illustrates further the positive effects of containing levels of expended energy and keeping them close to levels of perceived energy. On this day, fatigue ratings were in the moderate range (from 20 to 30) at the beginning of the day, while expended energy remained (undesirably) higher than perceived energy. At about 1:00

FIGURE 9.6

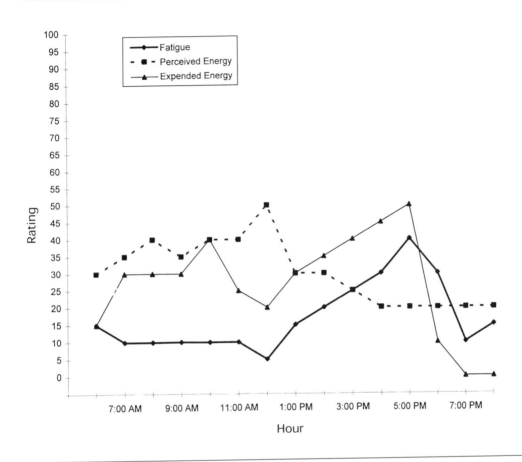

Hourly fatigue, perceived and expended energy for spring of 1995 (one example of initiation of a successful coping response).

p.m., this pattern reversed: Expended energy was consistently lower than perceived energy on almost every hourly rating. As a result, fatigue levels decreased gradually over the remainder of the day. Once again, keeping expended energy within the envelope of perceived energy yielded therapeutic reductions in fatigue.

In the fall of 1995, the participant's data patterns showed increased perceived energy and reduced fatigue (see Figure 9.8), in comparison with the data collected during the initial time period in the spring of 1995. Over the preceding months, the participant had made efforts to keep his expended energy close to his perceived energy. One can see the improving pattern of gradually increasing perceived and expended energy, with ratings of perceived and expended energy remaining relatively well matched.

FIGURE 9.7

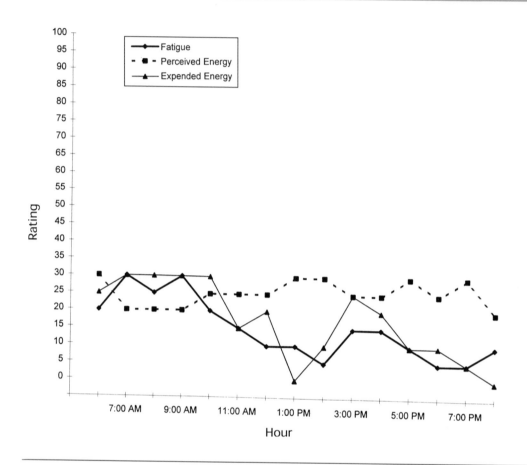

Hourly fatigue, perceived and expended energy for spring of 1995 (a second example of initiation of a successful coping response).

During the summer of 1996, 16 months after data collection had begun, a continuing improvement pattern is evident. In Figure 9.9, it is clear that the levels of fatigue (M =13%) are now considerably lower than the levels of perceived energy (M = 49%) and expended energy (M = 55%). The patient, by continuing his efforts to match perceived and expended energy, now showed a long-term reduction in fatigue as well as increased levels of perceived energy.

CLINICAL IMPLICATIONS OF ENVELOPE THEORY

Monitoring levels of expended energy, perceived energy, and fatigue over time appears to be a useful approach to the management of CFS.

FIGURE 9.8

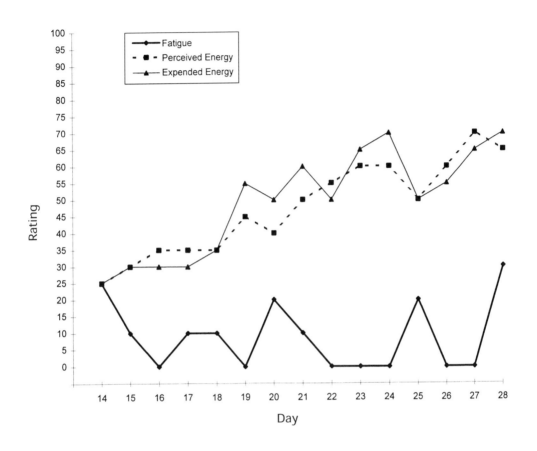

Daily fatigue, perceived and expended energy for fall of 1995.

Findings from the present case study demonstrate the critical relationship between expended energy, perceived energy, and fatigue for patients with CFS. When the participant's energy expenditure greatly exceeded his levels of perceived energy, fatigue levels were extremely high. In addition to exacerbating levels of fatigue, this overexertion also appeared to deplete the participant's energy resources. As the participant began to reduce expended energy to roughly his levels of perceived energy, fatigue levels remained low and perceived energy gradually increased. These findings show that levels of expended energy and perceived energy can be monitored and constructively balanced. The implications of this study are that people with CFS may be able to increase their energy resources while containing their levels of fatigue.

FIGURE 9.9

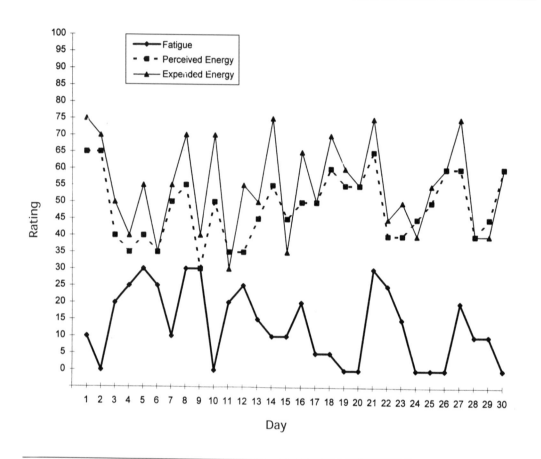

Daily fatigue, perceived and expended energy for summer of 1996.

With respect to clinical management, one of the most interesting findings involved the mediating role of perceived energy. Expended energy was associated with fatigue only when perceived energy was markedly exceeded. When expended energy increased gradually and did not greatly exceed perceived energy, fatigue was not exacerbated. Thus, when expended energy is maintained within the envelope of perceived energy, fatigue will lessen, and perceived energy will tend to be higher.

In the context of the current rest–activity debate, the results of the present study are instructive. Our data suggest that patients with CFS need to continuously monitor and assess their current levels of expended energy, perceived energy, and fatigue. For treatment plans to be as effective as possible, it is necessary that they be tailored to each individual and to his or her current condition.

Generating Coping Statements for the Patient

Our approach to cognitive coping is based on rational–emotive behavior therapy (Ellis, 1962, 1997; Ellis & Abrams, 1994). Specifically, stressful emotional reactions to CFS are assumed to be elicited by negative thoughts and beliefs that can be challenged and replaced with upset-reducing cognitive coping statements.

In CFS, the often encountered emotions of self-anger, guilt, and discouragement are related to negative evaluations of personal worth arising from CFS-related disability. Common self-denigrating thoughts in CFS are "I am weak" or "I am useless." Such global self-evaluations are amenable to the rational therapy model, which instructs clients to rate their behaviors rather than themselves. Specifically, clients are told that their activities (or lack of them) are not logically equivalent to a specific self-worth label—good or bad. Behaviors, on the other hand, can be rated or judged according to the client's value system. For example, a coping statement designed to counteract thoughts of self-rejection for a person with CFS might be "I am very frustrated by the things I can't do, but that does not make me weak or useless."

Although depression is the most commonly diagnosed psychological disorder in CFS (Friedberg, 1996a), discouragement or demoralization, a type of subclinical depression, may better characterize the emotional state of many of these patients who are strongly motivated to function better but cannot because of illness-related limitations (de Figueiredo, 1993; Ray, 1991).

> Demoralization may be viewed as a combination of distress and subjective incompetence. The main problem in demoralization is the sense of incompetence experienced by the demoralized individual; this sense of incompetence results from uncertainty as to the appropriate direction of action. By contrast, the major difficulty in endogenomorphic depression is a decreased magnitude of motivation even when the appropriate direction of action is known. (de Figueiredo, 1993, p. 308)

Discouragement or demoralization in CFS arises from the sense of reduced competence to manage vocational, marital, family, and social activities. Discouragement can have a profound effect on well-being, as the following narrative from a 45-year-old man with CFS suggests:

> Although I'm ill, I can still work part-time. But I still think about the things I can't do, like going out after work with friends or playing tennis more than once a month. Just that general feeling of being restricted from doing all the things I used to do. And that bad feeling grabs me whenever I think of doing something that I can't do now. Also, what gets to me is the exhaustion I feel

from just concentrating on work, even if I'm not putting forth much mental effort. I hardly ever feel good physically. And I react to this bad feeling, I now realize, with this creeping feeling of discouragement about the frustration of being restricted and never feeling quite right. What I'm learning, though, is that I can control this discouragement, which only worsens my feelings.

In addition to negative self-evaluations, low tolerance of frustration, the other major cause of emotional distress in the framework of rational therapy, is based on beliefs such as "It shouldn't happen," "I can't stand it," or "It's awful." The CFS patient might understandably endorse these beliefs as they consider their disabling symptoms, compared with pre-illness levels of functioning. Therefore, the client's right to endorse these views should be respected. Eventually, these stress-producing beliefs can be effectively disputed and replaced with coping statements that encourage tolerance of illness limitations and related problems.

Low frustration tolerance is commonly manifested in patients' beliefs that they should have total control of the illness. The patient may reason that they controlled their behavior before the illness and therefore should somehow be able to overcome their disability by sheer will. Clients may also believe that they should have such power or control because CFS is not a medically recognized illness. This mind–body cure notion has been strengthened by misleading mass media reports and popular psychology books (Hay, 1984; Siegel, 1986) that suggest chronic disabling illnesses can be ameliorated or even cured by single-minded determination, cognitive change, and lifestyle adjustments.

The therapist can emphasize the patient's ability to control attitude and behavior, rather than the totality of the illness. Simple questioning of the patient can effectively dispute the "total control" belief. The therapist may ask the client, "Why should you be able to completely control this illness? Where is the evidence?" Despite the persistence and intractability of their illness, patients may cling to the notion that they can fully maintain premorbid functioning. Although some people can sustain much of their pre-illness activity, others can do so only temporarily, or not at all. One CFS patient, a 26-year-old woman, described how she initially attempted to maintain premorbid functioning and the ruinous result:

> Before I got CFS, I worked a 50-hour-per-week sales job plus all my other activities. Despite my feelings of total collapse and fatigue when I became ill, I kept up with the job by drinking 10–12 cups of coffee a day. My apartment was a mess because I didn't have the energy to clean it up. I couldn't go out with friends or do anything else, because I had no energy. After a few months of this crushing schedule, I just collapsed. I knew then that I couldn't work. Looking back on it now, 2 years later, I see that I desperately

needed the rest. And I feel somewhat better now. I'm taking care of myself a lot better. It's been difficult with disability and all of that, but now I at least feel I can set up some goals for myself.

Fundamentally, therapeutic coping means that the clinician is helping the client adapt to the illness. *Adapt* or *tolerate* is preferable to the oft-used word *accept* as it applies to the restrictions of chronic illness. For many patients, *accept* implies surrender or giving up. *Adapt* or *tolerate* seems to have more constructive connotation. A four-stage model of psychological adjustment to CFS (see Appendix D; Fennell, 1995b) can be used by the clinician to help the client cope with the unpredictability of the illness. This model can reassure patients that their distress is an understandable reaction to a debilitating condition.

Coping With Disbelief

As previously stated, the disbelief of others about the reality of CFS is a major stressor for patients. Public and professional skepticism of the illness is based on (a) the absence of a biological marker or a diagnostic test to identify CFS, (b) the outwardly healthy appearance of many individuals with CFS (McKenzie et al., 1995) and (c) the extreme fluctuations in illness severity, which allow many patients to act normally one day only to plunge into a behavioral relapse the next (Friedberg et al., 1994). This variability in activity level may be interpreted by others as the patient's personal choice or simple malingering rather than uncontrollable manifestations of the illness. Disbelief may also be experienced by the family and friends of the patient who are feeling hurt, rejected, angry, or guilty about the loss of companionship and support associated with the ill person's limitations. This experience of loss may include a blaming of the individual with CFS for being ill (Fennell, 1995b; Register, 1987).

The patient's anger and hurt about others' open disbelief or even derision of their illness is a significant psychological issue. Anger may be intensified as patients futilely attempt to convince others, including physicians, that they are ill. It is important to allow expression of this anger in therapy sessions because it has not been well received by others. The clinician's understanding and tolerance of the anger is an important element of rapport building.

In social interactions, the problem of disbelief can begin with an ordinary "How are you?" Ask the patient how they handle such a routine inquiry. People with CFS usually learn to identify others who show genuine concern about their illness. However, on occasion, clients may get upset because they are expecting more concern and credibility than they receive. As an intervention, patients might be asked why it is important to convince others that they are ill with the goal of redirecting their efforts to network with supportive people and CFS-knowledgeable physicians, rather than to waste energy on skeptics.

A particular category of disbelief that the patient often encounters involves others' well-intentioned suggestions about home remedies, quick cures, and lifestyle adjustments for CFS. The general framework for such advice is "If you would just do X, you would be fine" (Friedberg, 1995c). Examples are "Look at the way you eat! Haven't you heard about the yeast-free diet?"; "You are so angry, just let it go"; "If I slept as much as you, I'd feel sick, too." The clinician can help the patient cope with this type of unsolicited advice through appropriate assertive skills. One humorous approach might be the following: If a family member suggests, "Why don't you take a nap if you are tired?" the patient might respond, "You know, that is such a good idea. I have not taken a nap since I have been ill and maybe that's the answer." Although this is a bit sarcastic, it indirectly conveys the frustration of the client to the skeptic without a useless verbal counterattack. Alternatively, the clinician can suggest to the client that they answer very directly, "Uncle Harry, I love you, but please don't give me advice about how to get well. I have tried so many remedies; it's just better for me if we talk about something else."

The treating clinician can also help the patient to understand the thinking of the skeptic. Healthy people may want to psychologically distance themselves from the chronically ill in an effort to believe that their health is not at risk (Fennell, 1995b; Friedberg, 1995c). To create that distance, the healthy person may believe that (a) there are ready solutions to an illness that the patient has not tried or (b) the ill person has done something wrong to deserve being ill, such as leading an unhealthy lifestyle. The distancing belief might be, "No, I would never do that thing that you did; therefore, I don't have to worry about getting a serious illness." With such self-reassuring ideas, the skeptic is able to cope with the threat of illness as presented by the patient, but unfortunately, at the patient's expense. Explaining the thinking of the skeptic to the patient may promote increased tolerance and fewer upsets about others' disbelief.

The Influence of Social Support on CFS

The skepticism and disbelief of others about the reality of CFS may be considered a type of "negative" social support that may significantly affect the emotional well-being of the ill person. Patients' level of functioning and their reactions to stress will be partially determined by the type of social and emotional support that they receive. Social support is a coping resource. Significant others can provide instrumental, informational, and emotional assistance (Thoits, 1995). Received social support promotes adjustment among people coping with illness possibly by facilitating reappraisal of uncertainty about the future (Mattlin, Wethington, & Kessler, 1990). A recent social support intervention for CFS patients (Schlaes & Jason, 1996) found that 1 hour per week of companionship and instrumental support and 2 hours per month of phone contact resulted in significant declines in fatigue severity and increases in positive thinking, while a control group experienced increases in fatigue severity and decreases in positive thinking. One client with CFS described his experience with a social support intervention as follows:

> I am really quite amazed by the positive impact that just talking to an understanding person has had for me. Although I am almost constantly fatigued, that feeling of being really connected was so enjoyable that it seemed to reduce my symptoms for a day or two afterwards. There really is a mind–body connection in this illness, not that CFS is all in your head, but that your emotions can affect the physical part of this illness.

A pilot study of marital social support in CFS (Schmaling & DiClementi, 1995) compared people with CFS who were in supportive marriages with those who were in unhappy, unsupportive marriages. Fatigue was moderately correlated with inactivity for CFS individuals in satisfied relationships, but it was not correlated with inactivity among patients in dissatisfied relationships. CFS participants in unhappy relationships were spending an average of nearly an hour a day more moving about and 30 minutes less reclining than were those individuals with CFS in satisfied relationships. These findings suggested that solicitous partners were inadvertently reinforcing disability. The lower activity levels in CFS participants in satisfied relationships suggest the utility of a clinical intervention: The additional sedentary time could have been more constructively focused on pleasant, nontaxing activities. Pleasant events have been associated with lower symptom severity and higher functioning in CFS (Ray et al., 1995b).

The findings of the Schmaling and DiClementi study suggest also that the individuals with CFS in dissatisfied relationships may have spent more time moving around than those in satisfied relationships because they received less physical support and relief from their partners. Although their function level was higher, the consequence of their increased mobility may have been more stress. Conversely, the

CFS-affected people in satisfied relationships may have been more satisfied (or less stressed) in part because they received physical assistance that allowed them more time for adequate rest.

The clinical issue raised by the above study concerns the possible reciprocal relationship between stress and functional status. Higher functioning compelled by the absence of social and physical support may not result in improved mood or happiness. On the other hand, the greater satisfactions associated with higher levels of support but lower functioning may limit the potential for constructive, low-effort activities. Ray, Weir, Phillips, and Cullen (1992) suggested that the opposing tendencies (as yielded in a factor analysis of CFS coping statements) of "maintaining activity" and "accommodating to the illness" are both used in CFS, depending on current energy level, environmental demands, social support, and so on. Rather than labeling "maintaining activity" as good and "accommodating to the illness" as bad, it may be more useful to evaluate each coping strategy as more or less appropriate to a particular situation or the patient's current symptom status.

Practical and emotional support for the CFS patient can range from stifling overprotectiveness at one extreme to persistent criticism and blame on the other. Overprotectiveness suggests that the patient's partner is assuming responsibility for completing activities and controlling the flow of information and news (Spacapan & Oskamp, 1992). This may create a helpless, out-of-control feeling in the spouse with CFS. A study of spousal support (Spacapan & Oskamp, 1992) confirmed that people who shielded their chronically ill partners from upsetting news or difficult decisions triggered feelings of being overprotected.

If overprotectiveness is an issue, the patient can be encouraged to have a frank and open discussion with his or her partner to identify the emotional triggers for the unwanted behavior. For instance, the healthy partner may resent the patient's disability or, on the other hand, derive satisfaction from caretaking. The patient's reactions to the overprotective behavior are also important. Does the patient think he or she is being controlled by the partner through unnecessary help or by buffering upsetting information? Such a conversation carried out with tact and sensitivity can lead to a plan to provide assistance to the patient at a mutually agreeable level. If the patient does not want the partner to withhold negative information and feelings, an assertive statement to that effect may help discourage the partner's overprotective inclinations.

Couples who are able to freely express their emotions about a spouse's chronic illness and its consequences have higher levels of marital satisfaction (Spacapan & Oskamp, 1992). In a recent study of marital relationships in 131 women with CFS (Goodwin, 1997), husbands who perceived themselves as empathic had wives who reported fewer symptoms. To moderate the healthy partner's feelings of over-responsibility for the ill person, it is also important for the patient to communicate to the partner that he or she does not have to solve all of the patient's problems but rather just listen and be supportive without judgment.

In contrast to the overprotective caregiver, the critical partner may be responding to personal frustrations, disappointments, and losses resulting from the ill person's limitations and symptoms. Once again, it is important for the person with CFS to engage the healthy partner in a discussion about his or her feelings about the illness. As specific emotions are articulated, then the attitudes and beliefs that sustain them can be identified. For instance, a healthy partner's anger may be related to the loss of companionship, sexual contact, and physical support as a result of the illness. Anger may also be fueled by disbelief that the person with CFS is really ill. Finally, the healthy partner's frustration may arise from the feeling of helplessness about the illness, especially when the patient complains about symptoms. Once these feelings are expressed, then a constructive negotiation may begin. The dissatisfied couple can be encouraged to make a list of items that they would like from each other followed by a negotiation to receive at least some of these items (e.g., sexual contact, affection, social outings).

To obtain a more comprehensive assessment of the patient's quality of social support, the Social Support Scale (Ray, 1992; see Appendix E) may be used. The scale is divided into 14 positive and 14 negative social support items. Scoring the test is less important than the specific information revealed about the social support environment of the patient. This information can be an important assessment tool in session.

Finally, two different types of verbalizations about CFS may be distinguished: (a) articulated feelings about the illness and its consequences and (b) expression of symptom complaints. It is usually stress-reducing for the patient to talk about the emotions associated with CFS. A tolerant partner will allow the patient to discharge these stressful feelings. On the other hand, persistent talking about CFS symptoms may encourage the patient to dwell on them excessively and alienate the healthy partner. Symptom complaints are appropriately expressed to a CFS-knowledgeable professional or another person with CFS who can best empathize with discussions about symptoms. The salutary effects of emotional disclosure have been summarized in a recent review (Pennebaker, 1995).

Memory Assistance

CFS patients report moderate to severe disturbances in memory and concentration and often consider these and other cognitive problems to be their most debilitating symptoms (Friedberg et al., 1994; Komaroff et al., 1996). Patients often report that their ability to think in a logical fashion can easily be derailed by a momentary distraction. In neuropsychological studies, the ability of people with CFS to shift from one mental task to another and then return to the original task is disrupted (DeLuca, Johnson, & Natelson, 1995). CFS-related work disability may be based on cognitive disturbance as well as impaired physical functioning.

The clinician can assist the cognitively impaired individual with CFS by first identifying emotional reactions to memory and concentration difficulties. These reactions may include self-anger, frustration, and discouragement. The client can then be told that getting frustrated and angry will only further impair their ability to stay focused and remember information. To minimize these disruptive emotional reactions, the strategies described herein may be helpful in coping with disruptive cognitive problems.

WORD BLOCK

Patients commonly report that they have difficulty retrieving specific words to convey a thought, complete a sentence, or simply carry on a conversation (Friedberg et al., 1994; Iger, 1992). A conversation may be halted by their frustrated attempt to recall a specific word or phrase. To reduce that type of frustration, clients may be advised that they do not have to pinpoint the exact words, but need only convey the idea, which can be expressed in other words. Patients can put together simple phrases that will bring them closer and closer to the idea they wish to convey. In addition, the listener can help the CFS individual's faltering speech. The listener may be willing to take some responsibility to help the patient through a difficult sentence or two or to ask questions that might revive the lost word or idea.

FORGETFULNESS

If forgetfulness is a major issue, visual cues can serve as reminders, such as writing notes in an established place where they can be easily found. A date book works nicely for some, or perhaps a clipboard in the car or a notepad or calendar on the refrigerator door.

If the patient forgets a particular plan or new idea, the lost memory may be retrieved. Suggest to the client, "Sit down, close your eyes, relax a moment and the thought may come back." If the client forgets where he or she put something, add these steps: "Visualize the situation leading up to the point of memory loss. Recreate the scene as faithfully as possible. For instance, if you have lost the car keys, sit down, relax, and visualize the last time you remember having them. Continue creating 'mental snapshots' leading forward in time until you identify the first scene in which you did not have the keys. Shift back and forth between scenes. These visualizations will assist recall." Tell the client it is more efficient to take mental snapshots than to turn the house upside down and get frustrated looking for a particular item.

COGNITIVE OVERLOAD

Finally, it is important for patients to avoid the overstimulation caused by too much activity based on a "do-everything" work ethic. Such compulsive behavior, physically tolerated prior to CFS onset, may now produce disabling cognitive symptom flare-ups. To reduce cognitive overstimulation, the following suggestions can be introduced by the treating clinician:

1. Allow extra time to complete activities. This will moderate symptom exacerbations and allow the client to mentally prepare for the next activity of the day.
2. Minimize distractions. For example, advise the client not to read with the radio on or attempt to balance a checkbook while others are in the room talking. Distractibility by noise (Friedberg et al., 1994) was ranked as the most frequent cognitive complaint in a large sample study of CFS.
3. Pattern daily activities into a routine that will minimize the stress on fragile cognitive capacities.
4. Break down all tasks and activities into incremental steps.
5. Focus only on step one until it is successfully completed before moving on to step two.
6. Watch for signs of increased mental fatigue and take necessary rest breaks.
7. Schedule relaxation techniques before studying, learning, or reading to reduce confusion and improve attention.

These practical suggestions to cope with cognitive overload are straightforward. However, lifestyle reductions to accommodate cognitive problems may be difficult for the patients to accept. Their potential resistance to these suggestions may be based on their desperate and often unsuccessful attempts to maintain a performance-based self-worth, for example, "I never had to write myself reminders and I don't want to start now!" The therapist is advised to use rational restructuring techniques (see pp. 159–161) to help the client distinguish the issues of self-worth and performance.

Conclusion

A number of cognitive–behavioral treatment techniques can be effectively focused on the symptoms and functional limitations in people with CFS. Clinicians can incorporate these interventions with their CFS patients and improve clinical outcomes. On the other hand, CFS researchers are faced with the divergence of clinical outcomes in published studies of cognitive–behavioral intervention, which may be explained by methodological differences as well as differences in patient characteristics. Current theoretical models that propose an association between stress and fatigue, and energy and fatigue (e.g., envelope theory) may have important implications for clinical treatment. As future behavioral treatments for CFS examine these variables, more definitive clinical recommendations can be made.

Clinical Interview With a CFS Patient   10

Because CFS patients usually present with symptoms of both medical and psychiatric illnesses, the clinician's task of assessment and treatment may be complicated. The following annotated clinical interview may be helpful in guiding the clinician's initial approach to the patient.

As CFS involves a wide spectrum of symptom severity and functional limitations, it is difficult to classify any patient as "typical." This case shows that even high-functioning individuals may have CFS. Although the patient presented herein is able to work full-time, albeit with great difficulty, many people with CFS are disabled from employment. For individuals with CFS who may work full-time, carry out selected family responsibilities, and perhaps do limited exercise, it seems implausible that schedules of increasing activity would yield a therapeutic benefit. Their behavioral pattern is one of working to exhaustion and collapsing afterward. This pattern is more amenable to an activity-pacing and stress reduction intervention (Friedberg & Krupp, 1994) rather than the graded activity schedules used with low-functioning clients (e.g., Deale et al., 1997).

The patient, Carolyn, is a 44-year-old psychiatrist, happily married for 23 years, with a 22-year-old son away at college. This initial psychological interview conducted by the first author (Friedberg) reveals the conflicts, dilemmas, and pervasive frustrations that are a consequence of CFS. Clinical observations are interspersed within the transcript to highlight important assessment issues (see chap. 7) that may become targets for subsequent treatment interventions (see chap. 9).

Therapist: You've seen several doctors for fatigue?

Patient: Yes. I saw a couple of doctors over the last 2 years. And whenever I talked about my complaints they looked at me like, "You need a psychiatrist." I guess I should treat myself. And then I stopped seeing anyone because no one paid any attention. When I saw the looks on their faces, I thought, What was the use for me to see them?

Therapist: What are the complaints that we're talking about?

Patient: I feel extremely tired and lethargic. Which is very unusual for me because I am a very active person. Before I became ill, I had a very active social life; I am still taking exercise classes. Whatever I'm doing, I'm moving fast, I'm talking fast . . . it's my personality. But I have periods of feeling exhausted, and then it's like I can't move.

Therapist: How many hours a week do you work?

Patient: I work 45 hours. I mostly see patients, but I also supervise residents treating their new patients.

Therapist: OK. In addition to work, you have had an active social life, and now you still exercise?

Patient: I used to take step classes, did the treadmill daily, and I went out a lot.

Therapist: You've had this very active lifestyle as long as you can remember?

Patient: Yes.

Therapist: And you found the lifestyle, as busy as it was, to be satisfying?

Patient: Yes, as it was.

Therapist: Did it seem to be too much at any point, or did it not?

Patient: No, no . . . I was very, very active.

Therapist: And you were happy about it?

Patient: Yes.

Therapist: Did you perhaps feel pressured or stressed by your job or anything else?

Patient: No, no . . . it might sound strange, because my job is stressful, but I really love my job. Second of all, I have excellent relationships with my coworkers. It's very unusual, but I have such good relationships that my job is like my second home.

Therapist: OK.

This patient is not acknowledging any distress about her highly active pre-morbid lifestyle, which included greater than full-time work, daily exercise, and social outings (as well as raising her son). By comparison, many CFS patients describe a hyperactive premorbid lifestyle involving work, family, social, and recreational activities that caused ongoing emotional distress and partial exhaustion states.

Patient: Third of all, I'm really enjoying my job because 2 years ago we started a new program, a course on treating personality disorders, which we have once every 3 months for 1 month. The course is led by two behavior therapists who are my friends, and I am learning from them how to do cognitive behavior therapy. I have learned how to manage my symptoms better.

Therapist: You mean the tiredness?

Patient: Yes. I think I know how to deal with this stress. But when my last chronic fatigue doctor told me, "Your job is stressful and you have to stop working for a couple of months," I said, "No, it's not my job that's causing this [CFS]." And then I didn't see her because I was scared.

Therapist: Scared of . . .

Patient: Of her suggestion not to work. And I decided, "I'm fine, I'm OK . . . ."

Therapist: Why did that suggestion scare you?

Patient: Because I would lose my mind *not* to work.

Therapist: OK.

Patient: Then I decided, I'm fine, I'm OK, like nothing's wrong with me. And all the tests were negative anyway. After I saw a couple of doctors and talked about my complaints and no one paid attention to me, my symptoms got progressively worse, up to the point that most of the time I'm tired and lethargic. If you divide all my time, I was basically OK 60% and not OK 40% of my time. Sometimes I'm a little bit better.

The patient was becoming upset by this line of questioning about stopping work. Although this is a significant clinical issue, the therapist decides, in the interest of rapport building, to return to basic diagnostic and assessment issues. A subsequent session, summarized at the end of this chapter, involved an important discussion of the work issue.

Therapist: Let me ask you more questions about your symptoms. Do you have problems with your memory or concentration since this illness began?

Patient: Yes. This is also very scary, because when the illness started, a couple of years ago, I could wake up and feel great and then suddenly feel so exhausted, that I did not feel like moving, and my concentration was terrible. It took me twice the time to do what is very easy for me. For example, when I feel this fatigue I have difficulty just looking at my appointment book to give an appointment. And I have to think very deliberately about what I'm doing when I feel like this.

Therapist: Are you also distractible?

Patient: Yes. And again, it's new to me. Because I'm usually very sharp.

Therapist: Is it like a very slowed down feeling mentally?

Patient: Yes.

Therapist: So you thought you could just manage a brief period of feeling lethargic.

Patient: Exactly.

Therapist: And just ignore it and go on with your work, but the feeling has become more and more intrusive.

Patient: It got progressively worse up to the point that I can only manage working. I don't have a social life.

Therapist: Why not?

Patient: Because I have to be in bed. Even after having 8 hours of sleep, I never feel refreshed. I'm always waking up, and I don't feel like I've gotten a good night's sleep. But if I'm sleeping at least 8 hours I'm able to function the next day. All of my efforts are directed toward being able to function. I'm not going out socially, because I have to be in bed. If I'm not in bed at 10:00 or 10:20 it's extremely difficult for me to function the next day. That is how I live, kind of around my symptoms.

Therapist: Have you taken any vacations away since all of this started?

Patient: What do you mean?

Therapist: Vacations away from this general area.

Patient: No, I did not take vacations, but when I feel like this it doesn't make any difference.

Therapist: I'm not necessarily talking about stress or the absence of it when you go on vacation. Just a change of environment.

Patient: I see. I went to Canada and to Lake George for 7 or 10 days....

Therapist: When you were at Lake George for a week, you didn't feel any better at the end of the week than at the beginning?

Patient: No.

Therapist: What were you doing up there that week?

Patient: You know, we kind of walked around and rested, we rented a small house in the woods.

Therapist: No major physical activity? You weren't reading technical books or . . . anything like that?

Patient: No. And you know, the rest was not helping me. I didn't feel better. I spent a whole day doing nothing. And I didn't feel better, I felt worse. Like I had wasted a whole day.

Therapist: You mean you felt worse on an emotional level.

Patient: Mentally, yeah. When I feel like this, I'm still trying to do something, or to fix something, or like . . . to read a fashion magazine or rent a movie. Because resting is not helping me. When I feel so tired and lethargic, nothing helps, nothing at all. Just 2 weeks ago, I felt this fatigue 3 or 4 days in a row. It's such an awful feeling. I walk around the house. It's not like I have a fever and lying in the bed might help me. Lying in the bed, I feel worse. I try to read, I try to go outside, I try to take a walk, I try to play with my dog. I try to do something. I'm just trying to be functional.

The patient's symptom status during nonworking vacations or intervals where responsibilities were significantly reduced is an important diagnostic issue. If symptoms rapidly decline during these periods, the patient may have non-CFS chronic fatigue, a condition that can respond much more rapidly to coping skills, such as activity pacing and stress reduction. On the other hand, when restful time off does not yield substantial symptom reductions, then an assessment for full-blown CFS is warranted.

Therapist: What used to be routine is now an effort.

Patient: Yes.

Therapist: Let me ask you a few other questions. Are you getting headaches?

Patient: Yes.

Therapist: Since this all began, is it a new type of headache?

Patient: Yes, because I have a history of migraine headaches, for many, many years. But I have learned how to manage it; before a migraine headache I usually feel a throbbing sensation over my eyes, but my Fiorinol relieves the headache. And then I started to have unusual headaches. I can't even describe it.

Therapist: The new headaches, are they pressure-like?

Patient: Pressure-like, yes.[1]

Therapist: OK. Do you still get the migraines?

Patient: Yeah.

Therapist: How often?

Patient: Oh, not too often. Once every 2 to 3 weeks. But the Fiorinol does not help the new type of headache.

Therapist: How severe is this headache, the new type of headache?

Patient: Not severe, but very bothering and prolonged.

Therapist: OK. Joint pains?

Patient: No.

Therapist: Flu-like symptoms?

Patient: No.

Therapist: Swollen glands?

Patient: No, no . . .

Therapist: How about muscle pain?

Patient: Just some muscle pain when I go upstairs.

Therapist: OK. Muscle weakness?

Patient: Sometimes, yes. Especially, when I started to take step classes, which I really love doing, because I love dancing. And after taking the classes I could, like, move mountains I felt so good. I went out, I did something at home, I played with the dog. And then one and a half years ago I noticed something, I felt tired after classes. And my muscles ached. After exercising I didn't feel better, I felt worse.

Therapist: All right. Any stomach, intestinal or bowel problems?

Patient: None of those.

Therapist: OK. Any medical or physical problems before age 30?

Patient: No. I was quite healthy back then.

At this point, the therapist has asked Carolyn about each symptom listed in the case definition of CFS (Fukuda et al., 1994; see Exhibit 1.1). Because the patient reports more than 6 months of persistent, medically unexplained fatigue not alleviated by rest, plus five out of eight secondary symptoms (unrefreshing sleep, exercise intolerance, cognitive difficulties, new type of headache, muscle weakness), she meets criteria for CFS.

---

[1]It appears that pressure-like headaches are the most commonly reported type of headaches in CFS.

The patient's complaints are not consistent with a diagnosis of somatization disorder, which requires a significant history of physical complaints before age 30. In addition, symptom criteria for somatization disorder include at least four types of pain symptoms, two gastrointestinal symptoms, one sexual symptom, and one pseudoneurologic symptom. The patient reports only one pain symptom (headache) and no gastrointestinal symptoms. She did describe a pseudoneurologic symptom, muscle weakness, but this problem is a postexercise complaint that is closely associated with CFS. In a subsequent session, she revealed a loss of sexual desire, a common complaint in CFS, that may also be considered a somatization symptom. However, given the absence of a history of somatization complaints, it would seem more plausible to classify the sexual symptom as a consequence of a severely fatiguing illness.

As CFS is defined by self-report symptom criteria, the mental health clinician can verify a CFS diagnosis and then determine how these symptoms affect functioning and well-being. CFS symptom overlap with clinical depression and generalized anxiety disorder is discussed later in this chapter.

Therapist: How about the day after the exercise. How do you feel?

Patient: Ah, so-so.

Therapist: No worse?

Patient: No. [*Note: CFS patients often* do *report symptom flare-ups 24 hours after exercise.*] I still exercise, but I'm not exercising for an hour every morning on the treadmill like I used to. I'm exercising for 20 minutes, but not as often as before, perhaps twice a week on Saturdays and Sundays.

Therapist: Do you feel good during the exercise, or not even that?

Patient: I'm pushing myself. I strongly believe in an active lifestyle, which is why I'm not someone who is giving up. Before, when I exercised it was such fun, I looked forward to it. Right now I am not looking forward to it. Not at all. I'm just doing it because I feel that it's very important. You know, like I'm pushing myself.

Therapist: Why do you do two exercise classes on the weekend but none during the weekdays?

Patient: Because it's very difficult when I get home after work. I'm exhausted. I feel like collapsing. When I come home I feel like going straight from my car to my bedroom, like not even going through the hall and kitchen....

Therapist: Do you ever dwell on your symptoms?

Patient: Just the opposite. I ignore my symptoms. I always say I'm OK even when I feel horrible.

The absence of symptom preoccupation is quite consistent with Carolyn's presentation as a determined, single-minded, work-oriented individual who copes with the illness by trying to deny it as much as possible. Although denial coping is associated with greater stress (Friedberg et al., 1994) and impairments (Antoni et al., 1994) in CFS, it appears to contradict a central assumption of the symptom avoidance model that functional impairments are driven by a fear of exacerbating symptoms. In contrast, this patient pushes herself until she collapses from exhaustion.

Therapist: OK. Do you feel depressed about all of this, or not?

Patient: No, I don't feel depressed in general.

Therapist: Or do you feel a loss of interest?

Patient: I don't have a loss of interest. I am not doing my activities because I can't. I don't have a loss of interest in anything. But unfortunately, what I feel is that I'm not living, only surviving. Before, I lived a very full life.

Therapist: If not a loss of interest, do you have a loss of enjoyment in doing things that would normally be satisfying?

Patient: Yes. When I'm severely fatigued, I can function to some extent, but I don't feel enjoyment.

Therapist: How often do you feel so fatigued that you can't enjoy what you do?

Patient: About 50% of the time.

Clearly, the patient is experiencing a loss of pleasure or anhedonia when her fatigue is severe. The question is whether the CFS symptom exacerbation triggered a reactive anhedonia, a preexisting anhedonic state increased fatigue, or the CFS produced both increased fatigue and the inability to experience pleasure. If the fatigue exacerbations are a consequence of physical and mental exertion or stress, as would be confirmed by a stress symptom log, then stress reduction and pacing interventions (see chap. 9) would be beneficial. If the anhedonia is associated with melancholic depression, then pleasant mood induction, possibly in combination with antidepressant medication, might be helpful.

Therapist: Do you feel demoralized?

Patient: No, but you have to know me, I'm very strong. I'm not letting myself feel probably what people should feel in this situation.

Therapist: Why is that?

Patient: Why, because I fight.

Therapist: To let yourself feel demoralized, would that be like giving in?

Patient: Yes, because I've gone through a lot of stress in my life. I lost my parents at a young age. And I was in a bad car accident just before I was to start my residency training. So, I'm not just giving up.

Therapist OK.

Patient: When I feel like this, severely fatigued, I feel down. But I feel down from being fatigued. I don't feel depressed, like down in the dumps, or whatever. I feel like I really want to do something, but it's very difficult for me to plan anything. Like going out. Because it's happened many times when we planned to go somewhere and then suddenly I felt so lethargic and tired that I felt like fainting in the car. And we had to go home. A couple of times, I almost lost consciousness behind the wheel, because I felt so lethargic. My concentration level dropped and I started to lose track of where I was on a road I had taken many times.

Therapist: How about feelings of diminished self-esteem or worthlessness?

Patient: No.

Therapist: Changes in weight or appetite?

Patient: Because I'm not exercising like I did before, yes, I put on 8, maybe 10 pounds, since last year. But even if I'm eating very healthy, eating fruits and vegetables, basically all the time, I put on weight because I'm not as active as before.

Therapist: Is that upsetting?

Patient: Upsetting? . . . I don't like it. Because I care about my appearance.

The patient reports four out of the five symptoms required for a diagnosis of major depression (DSM-IV): concentration difficulty, persistent fatigue, unrestful sleep, and periods of anhedonia (associated with severe fatigue). As is typical in CFS patients, Carolyn reports no loss of interest in doing activities. Although these symptoms might suggest a subclinical depression, we would argue that these symptoms are more likely to be manifestations of CFS (see chap. 7). First, the fatigue symptom itself is reported to be intense and disabling, which is more characteristic of CFS than of depression. Second, her concentration problems are so severe that she cannot drive or read attentively for more than a few minutes. Once again, the intrusiveness of this symptom appears to be far greater than what would be expected for clinical depression. Third, the loss of enjoyment is present only during unpredictable bouts of severe fatigue. When loss of enjoyment is a feature of clinical depression, it is persistent and pervasive and is typically worse in the morning. Finally, her sleep disturbance, which involves numerous nighttime awakenings, cannot be easily categorized as a CFS or a depression symptom because this specific type of sleep pattern has not been addressed in the research literature. In sum, we believe that the patient's symptom reports are more consistent with CFS than syndromal depression.

Therapist: Do you tend to worry about things?

Patient: Not to an extreme. Yeah, I do, like all human beings, but not in an extreme way, not obsessive with worry.

Therapist: Any particular worries that recur?

Patient: Yeah, what will happen to the hospital where I work. The hospital is not making money, and jobs may be lost.

Therapist: Oh, I see.

Patient: I'm a survivor, I'm a fighter. And I'm using different techniques in order to be able to survive and not give up. When I have concerns, I'll worry for a couple of hours, until the evening, and the next morning I'll be doing what needs to be done.

Therapist: So you might worry for a couple of hours in the evening about something.

Patient: If something comes up . . . you know, whatever issue. . . .

Therapist: The reason I'm asking is because if you worried occasionally for a couple of hours in the evening before this illness started, you just slept through the night and were fine the next day. Now if you worry, it may take its toll on you physically, because you may be much more stress-sensitive than you were. You probably have a certain vulnerability to stress now you didn't have before, both emotional and physical. So you don't tolerate the stress as well, even the emotional stress, which may have a more subtle effect than the more obviously draining physical exertion.

Patient: You're probably right.

Therapist: So, as a result, your fatigue can increase subtly and gradually over time for emotional reasons you're not even aware of.

Patient: OK, I understand what you're talking about.

Therapist: One thing I can help you with is managing that type of stress and becoming more aware of how it affects your symptoms.

In CFS patients, low-level emotional stresses, such as discouragement, irritability, mild persistent anxiety, and minor frustrations may increase or magnify CFS symptoms so that the illness becomes more intrusive and debilitating. Yet the patient may not associate emotional stress with CFS symptoms. The therapist can educate the patient through assigned daily record forms to chart stress and symptom fluctuations. Then coping-oriented cognitive–behavioral techniques (see chap. 9) such as relaxation, pleasant mood induction, and activity pacing can be taught to counteract the unhealthy stress–symptom interactions.

Therapist: Do you experience anxiety?

Patient: Yes. But it's not like a continuous thing. If I hear the phone ring, I get palpitations. Any sudden noise might do that. And it takes me a while to calm down. Before I got sick, I had low-level anxieties, but they kind of helped me, spurred me on. Now with the illness, I get these startle-like reactions. I sometimes feel like I'm going to fall apart.

Therapist: OK. Do you feel restless or keyed up or on edge?

Patient: No.

Therapist: How about irritability?

Patient: In general, no.

Although Carolyn reports occasional worries, in particular a realistic fear about losing her job or being unable to work, she does not meet the two principal criteria for generalized anxiety disorder: excessive and difficult-to-control anxiety or worry lasting for at least 6 months. The patient does meet secondary criteria for generalized anxiety disorder, including easy fatigability, difficulty concentrating, and sleep disturbance. However, the severity of these debilitating symptoms is more consistent with CFS. (Her hyperreactivity to noise is a commonly reported complaint in CFS.) Perhaps the critical difference between CFS and generalized anxiety disorder is that the fatigue symptom in CFS is predominant, severe, and disabling, whereas the fatigue associated with generalized anxiety disorder is usually subordinate to intense, ongoing anxiety or worry. The important clinical issue is the effect of her worry and distress on her physical functioning and emotional well-being.

Patient: OK. Also, what I wanted to tell you is one of the reasons I am able to survive is because of my family, because of my husband. I have a very good family. And my husband is doing everything. He is driving me back and forth, he's cooking, he's shopping, he's doing the laundry, he's taking care of the house, the dogs, he's doing everything. In this way, I am able to work because I am able to concentrate on what needs to be done in order to be able to work.

The complex issue of social support and related decisions about work in CFS is well illustrated here. Carolyn's husband, by doing the bulk of the housework, allows her to endure a 45-hour work week. Yet the patient's condition is worsening, which may plausibly be related to her workload. The family requires the income, but if her husband did not drive her to work and maintain the house, she might be compelled to stop working and apply for disability. Her husband could return to work if necessary.

A temporary work termination might permit her to schedule fewer activities with more flexibility and to facilitate some level of symptomatic improve-

ment. Then, she could work a small number of hours, say, in private practice. However, she is not board-certified as a psychiatrist, a significant hindrance to successful practice in a managed care environment. She felt unable to prepare adequately for a board certification test because her ability to read and retain information was significantly impaired by the illness. Also, the patient has rejected this possibility because she loves her work, as it is.

Often, people with CFS will force themselves to work until the illness becomes severely disabling. The clinician may offer assistance by outlining, in collaboration with the patient, all of the work and activity options that are feasible. This process of carving out viable work and nonwork options may lessen the anxiety about losing the ability to continue a current job.

For many individuals with CFS, the decision to continue working or to stop working and, if necessary, apply for disability benefits is an excruciating dilemma. On one hand, continuing to work preserves what may be a satisfying job and the self-esteem associated with it. But the psychological cost is high: The physical and mental exertion of work may cause worsening of the illness while depleting limited energies for other important activities, including marital, family, social, and recreational pursuits. If the patient chooses to continue working, stress reduction techniques may be the most helpful intervention.

On the other hand, terminating employment may offer a better chance for recovery or improvement in CFS, while allowing greater attention to other important activities. Yet one's sense of personal value may be diminished and the difficult process of redefining purpose and direction may take years to accomplish. The clinician can assist the patient in articulating these alternatives in order to make better informed decisions about major lifestyle changes and adjustments.

Therapist: So before, you were sharing the household responsibilities and now you just have to focus all of your attention on work because that is all you can do?

Patient: No, I am still doing something at home, because I just can't *not* do it. Then, when I do it I feel a little bit better. For days or weeks at a time I can only work. But when I feel a little bit better, I'm trying to catch up with other things. When I feel better I am trying to do something which does not even need to be done, because I don't know when I'll feel worse again. Make sense?

Therapist: Yes. When you feel good, you want to make up for all the things you couldn't do.

Patient: The problem is that I never feel good. I may feel fatigued or I may feel better.

Therapist: OK. But never good.

Patient: Almost never. I can't remember the last time when I felt good.

Therapist: When this all started a couple of years ago, was it sudden or was it a gradual thing?

Patient: I think it was gradual. I remember clearly when it started for the first time, I felt so lethargic and fatigued, which is very unusual for me. I clearly remember this scary episode. When I went to a doctor, who I know is a very good doctor, he told me, "Oh, don't worry, it's nothing terrible. . . ." Like I told you. And he's a very knowledgeable doctor. He did all kinds of tests, everything was OK. So I decided, OK, I have to learn how to live with this.

Therapist: Well, that may or may not be true, that you have to live with this. Some people do recover from this. Most people say they feel somewhat better over time; but not too many people say they have completely recovered.

Patient: Do you see people like me, where it's getting progressively worse?

Therapist: I have. About a third will say they get worse over time. You're into this only 2 years.

Patient: No, more.

Therapist: Oh, it is more than 2 years?

Patient: The symptoms started intermittently maybe 4 or 5 years ago. Two years ago it got progressively worse. When it started, I had periods of extreme lethargy maybe for 6 or 8 hours once in a week, once in 2 weeks, not often. And again, when it just started, intially I was scared, because I didn't know what it was. But then, I began to realize that it would get better the next day. And I was able to overcome it by being able to figure out my priorities, and doing only what was necessary that day. But I knew that the next day I would feel better, because these periods were very short.

Therapist: Oh, I see.

Patient: And again 2 years ago, one of the doctors asked me, "Do your coworkers know about it?" and I said, "No." And she was very surprised. "How come, when you feel like this?" And I said, because I am able to cover up, because I just smile, and don't show how I feel, because I don't like anyone to know that I don't feel well. And I don't like people to feel sorry for me. Sometimes, I feel like going home, closing my eyes, putting shades on the window, and not talking to anyone, but I continue to work. And what I have learned is that, no matter how I feel, I just smile. And if anyone asks how I am, I say I'm fine, I'm OK.

Therapist: There's no good reason to tell anyone other than people very close to you. I mean, what can they do?

Patient: I don't like to complain. When I feel like this, I talk a little to myself, thinking it's nothing that terrible and that tomorrow or the day after tomorrow I'll feel better. I'll be thinking, like, I'll be able to perform.

Therapist: "It's not so bad."

Patient: Yes. I've learned how to think positively. For example, at work I left early one day, which is very unusual for me . . . usually whenever I don't feel well, even if I have a fever, I never leave a couple of hours early. I never call in sick. I have accumulated a lot of sick days and vacation days because I know my responsibilities. I have 120 patients and I know everyone at the hospital is working hard. I cannot call in sick because someone has to do my job. But recently I felt so bad that at 2:00 I just had to go home. I had a severe migraine headache. And I called my husband and he picked me up.

   Before I got sick I woke up in the morning and did laundry, or exercised on the treadmill or I went outside with the dog . . . and now I'm dragging myself. It takes me more than one hour to take a shower and get dressed. My husband is cooking lunch, while I have learned how to take a "medical" shower. I rapidly change the water from hot to cold and back. So I take a very, very cold shower for seconds, minutes, as much as I can tolerate. Now that I'm taking such a cold shower, I'm able to open my eyes, you know, and comb my hair and get dressed and move myself out of the house.

Therapist: I'm impressed. Drastic measures, but I guess they work. Do you do any type of self-relaxation or meditation?

Patient: No.

Therapist: Do you have trouble relaxing?

Patient: Yes. I do. I'm beginning to think relaxation might be a good thing for me. But just sitting and relaxing seems so unproductive.

Therapist: I can show you relaxation techniques that you can do easily and quickly. And I think that once you experience a deeply relaxed feeling, you'll feel better about taking that time.

Patient: Now, when I feel bad I distract myself and think about something pleasant. When I'm feeling really exhausted I think positively. I'll go home and I'll see my two dogs and on the weekend I'll be able to spend time with my son and my husband and I will go to the movies. So I'm distracting myself this way. I think I can write a book, you know, on how I'm learning to survive.

The patient is practicing pleasant mood induction, a technique that can not only distract from symptoms, but uplift mood, reduce symptom severity, and, according to a prospective study (Ray et al., 1995b) lead to long-term improvements.

Therapist: It sounds good. That's what I do, teach coping skills for problems. OK. Do you and your son get along very well?

Patient: Yeah, we have a very good relationship.

Therapist: Now in general, I think these coping skills that you're using are helpful, more or less. What I can offer you is the coping skills that you have not learned yet, and that you could benefit from, like relaxation and managing emotional stress better.

Patient: OK.

Therapist: There are different things that I will examine in relation to the illness and your lifestyle. I'm sure you've done a lot of self-examination on how to pace yourself and conduct your lifestyle in a way that's going to make you feel as functional as possible. But it's still a major exercise in frustration with this illness. Do you have any questions for me?

Patient: No, I'm listening. Whatever help you can offer I'd be more than happy because I don't think I'm living. I'm very strong and I'm a fighter, and I know how to make myself feel better. I'm always taking care of myself and I would never go to my job without my proper makeup and my hair done and dress properly, which is why my friends can't believe I have chronic fatigue syndrome. One friend, who's a psychiatrist, told me he was upset to hear I was ill. I said, why? He told me I am like an example for him all the time because I am very active and usually smiling, and such a good doctor. He couldn't believe that I didn't feel good and he didn't notice it. And I told him, don't worry, it's OK because I know how to control it. But I'm not doing much else than work.

Therapist: Well, your work life is very important to you, so you'll sacrifice as much as you can in order to keep your work life going.

Patient: And my social life is also important.

Therapist: But in a sense you've prioritized, to say that work is really the more important of those two things.

Patient: Mmmm ... I don't know. My relationship with my husband is also important, and ... we don't have a life.

Therapist: You have only so many hours that you can do some meaningful, purposeful work. Clearly, you're maintaining your 45 hours of work.

Patient: Just ...

Therapist: Hanging by a thread I guess. OK, let's say you wake up every day with x amount of energy.

Patient: I don't have energy.

Therapist: Well, let's put it this way: You're running on something. Something is getting you through the day. Maybe you don't call it energy, but it's something. And you're getting worse, which suggests that the amount of energy you are using up may be more than you have, considerably more. Now you have a fraction of the energy you used to have. If your activities always far exceed the energy you have, you will exhaust yourself and your illness may worsen over time. If you keep the two in balance, [the energy you have (perceived energy) and the energy you use up (expended energy)], you may stabilize your condition, and over time you might even get a little better. But of course that involves a lot of tough decisions that you probably don't want to make. For instance, you want to keep the job because you like it so much.

[The constructs of perceived energy and expended energy are based on an emerging concept of energy conservation in CFS, the envelope theory (see chap. 9).]

Patient: I'm not trying to make any drastic decisions. But I'm taking one day at a time and I have learned how to divide my day by hours. I'm not thinking that I have to work until 4:00. I'm thinking, you have to work until 12:00. Then from 1:00 to 4:00 ... I'm dividing the days by hours.

Therapist: That's fine, that's fine. Don't put any unnecessary pressure on yourself. Just say: "I'll take it one hour at a time." But the mental exertion of being at work is an enormous drain on you because you're ill.

Patient: I would be happy to work less but it's not an option.

Therapist: That's the other thing ... if you could ...

Patient: It's 45 hours or nothing.

Therapist: Really? OK. That's if you want to stay there.

Patient: Yes . . . not just for psychiatrists. I don't know if you know this, but it's not an option. The option is to work the 45 hours or not to work. And another reason is that my coworkers, my colleagues sacrifice and are very helpful. If I need something I don't have to ask twice. I don't have to ask for it. People were offering me help before I told them I have chronic fatigue syndrome. Because I have such a good relationship with everyone. That is why it is very good for me to work.

Therapist: You're lucky. You have a very supportive environment at work and at home. But all that support kind of allows you to exhaust yourself every day.

Patient: And again, I'm not living. Well, I feel a little bit better talking about this . . . . Can I ask you something?

Therapist: Yes.

Patient: Ahh . . . is it possible that it might get worse up to the point that . . . OK . . . might get worse than it is?

Therapist: Yes, it may. You're just functioning on pure gumption you could say, pure guts and nerve, rather than physical stamina. I understand that this is a major fear, getting worse. And the idea that you're giving up if you do less than you do. These are important issues that I can help you with.

The Axis I diagnostic impression for this patient is adjustment disorder with mixed emotional features, rather than syndromal depression or anxiety. Carolyn is also experiencing enormous job-related stress. Although a thorough assessment of personality pathology was not done, a clinician could reasonably argue for the presence of at least one obsessive–compulsive personality trait characterized by "excessive devotion to work and productivity to the exclusion of leisure activities and friendships (not accounted for by obvious economic necessity)" (*DSM-IV*).

The treatment plan for this patient involved (a) increased awareness of emotional stress and its effect on symptoms; (b) prescribed self-relaxation for stress reduction, improved well-being, and more restful sleep; and (c) constructive reevaluation of working commitments in light of worsening illness. (The patient had previously refused medication, other than Fiorinol for migraines, for symptom management and was still unreceptive to it.)

Over several therapy sessions, Carolyn showed progress toward the first two goals; however, she initially rejected any alternatives to her current work schedule (goal three). In Sessions 2 and 3, she was taught breathing-focus relaxation (see chap. 9), which was incorporated into her daily work schedule. As a result, she began to recognize the connection between the ongoing stress of work and increased CFS symptoms. The relaxation exercise provided an important feeling of relief from this symptom stress and generated a sense of improved well-being. Because she rarely felt "good," the relaxation-enhanced improvement in her feeling state was an important therapeutic benefit.

During Session 5, the patient revealed that a previous discussion about suspending work and applying for disability compensation initially made her very nervous. On further reflection, she could view temporary disability as a practical option that would eliminate the physical and emotional exertion of daily work and perhaps facilitate improvements in her illness. She expressed relief just to believe that she had an alternative to work. The patient also began to recognize that her persistent efforts to "fight" the illness by maintaining a damaging workload were a form of denial rather than a constructive coping strategy.

As she incorporated stress-reducing techniques into her daily schedule, she felt a somewhat heightened ability to endure her long work week. After eight therapy sessions over a 6-month period, she declared, "I will work until I can't work." She explained this decision by saying that she now recognized the unhealthy aspects of demanding full-time work and would apply for disability if it became physically impossible for her to keep her job. The patient's resolution reflected a greater recognition and acceptance of her current conflicts and a viable plan if her work could not be sustained.

Was this decision a healthy one, given her gradually deteriorating physical condition? Perhaps it was not. Would it have been more constructive to take a medical leave from work to allow time for rest, improvement, or possibly recovery? In the therapist's view, a 1-year suspension from work would have been the more desirable alternative. But the patient's motivation to work superseded all other considerations. As in any therapeutic endeavor, the ultimate decisions are made by the patient. In this case, Carolyn completed the course of treatment with important insights and coping skills, although her illness condition remained little changed.

An Eight-Session Coping Skills Treatment Program for CFS Groups

11

The first author (Friedberg) has conducted several fatigue and stress management groups for CFS patients based on cognitive–behavioral principles. Therapy group outcome data for a coping skills approach to CFS were reported in a published study (Friedberg & Krupp, 1994). A standardized protocol, developed for a CFS group intervention, is summarized herein. The techniques prescribed are referenced to detailed instructions in chapter 9. The treatment regimen may be adapted to an individual therapy format as well.

Session 1

Initially, patients are asked to complete a brief self-report psychological assessment, including (a) the Beck Depression Inventory (BDI), a 21-item self-report measure of depression symptoms; (b) the Beck Anxiety Inventory, a 21-item measure of anxiety; (c) the Fatigue-Related Cognitions Scale, a 14-item assessment of fatigue-related thinking (see Appendix C; Friedberg & Krupp, 1994); and (d) the Fatigue Severity Scale, a 9-item measure of the effect of fatigue on functioning (Krupp et al., 1989). These self-report instruments may be more sensitive to treatment changes in patients with higher levels of comorbid depressive symptomatology (Friedberg & Krupp, 1994).

Following completion of these self-report assessments, the clinician presents a synopsis of the therapy format and goals. Participants are told that they will be able to share their feelings about having CFS in a supportive, nonjudgmental milieu, and will be asked specific questions about the illness by the therapist in an effort to understand their difficulties. Interaction among the participants is encouraged. The therapeutic emphasis is on (a) improvement of psychological coping skills, (b) practical suggestions for illness-related issues, and (c) behavioral home assignments.

INTRODUCTION TO THE FIRST SESSION

The following overview of the treatment program is given to patients:

> Chronic fatigue syndrome is a poorly understood, debilitating illness. The stress of the illness and its impact on your lifestyle can be overwhelming. Discouragement and frustration will arise from many sources, including marital, financial, and vocational strains as well as the stress of the illness itself. You will get help here to deal with these stressors. First of all, you will receive support, a sense of feeling understood by others who have the same illness. Second, we will talk about coping techniques. Coping techniques can restore a sense of control. Anything you can do for yourself that restores a sense of control is a profound aid.
>
> We will deal with a number of illness issues, including the limitations on what you can do, the stress created by the illness, the unpredictability of symptoms, the difficulty in planning to do things, and the disbelief of others who may think the illness is all in your head. Also, we will discuss how to maintain a good relationship with your spouse or partner, or if that isn't possible, how to cope with a difficult relationship. You can develop new ways of communicating clearly about your feelings, expectations, and desires, such as being able to say, "I need your help now." You can also learn how to be assertive in dealing with doctors and bureaucratic systems.
>
> If you identify with your job, or your role as a spouse or parent, you may feel diminished or worthless when you can no longer do these things as well as you did. You can learn to be more flexible about the image you have of yourself and realize that self-esteem is a question of who you are, and not what you do. We will deal with the fear of becoming indulgent and useless. This is not an illness to die of, but because it is still incurable, CFS has become an illness to live with. You can learn to live with it better than you may realize.

STRUCTURED ACTIVITIES

Initially, participants will state their first name, followed by a self-description of their illness, including its duration, current symptoms, and debilitating effects. To encourage disclosure of emotional reactions to the illness, participants are asked what they have lost because of the illness (e.g., ability to work, friends) and how it has affected their lives. The answers to this question will help the therapist understand how each individual is coping with these losses. Coping reactions can range from one behavioral extreme of denial, which may involve a desperate and often self-damaging effort to retain pre-illness functioning, to the other extreme of severe vegetative depression, where the patient feels helpless and immobilized. Revelations about emotional reactions to CFS will facilitate a group interchange based on nonjudgmental understanding, constructive suggestions, and a sense of shared coping. This exercise may help initiate the difficult process of emotional and behavioral adaptation to illness-related losses.

Once the issue of illness losses is fully aired, the stressful aspects of social interaction may be introduced. The clinician asks patients how they respond to the routine "how are you's" from others: To whom can they answer truthfully? Are they expecting more concern than they actually receive from family and friends? Do discussions about their illness result in unsolicited advice from others that further frustrates the patient? How do they react to the often-heard statement, "But you look so good!"? The discussion of social encounters highlights the dramatic, and usually negative changes that have taken place in interpersonal relationships because of the disabling effects of CFS. For instance, friendships may be strained, and family members may be unsupportive, critical, or skeptical. Cognitive reevaluation techniques to reduce the emotional distress of social encounter can then be introduced.

Patients are then asked to describe any encounters with friends, family, doctors, or even total strangers in which they have gotten the message to "heal yourself." How did they feel about it? (See pp. 161–162 for further information on skepticism about the illness and how patients can understand, cope with, and respond to such advice.)

To provide a break in the emotional intensity provoked by the preceding questions, the next suggested topic involves prior treatments tried by the participants. What successes or failures have they experienced in their efforts to find help for their illness? This discussion may lead to an important and potentially helpful exchange of information about medical and alternative therapies. A list of patient-rated treatments for CFS is available (see Figure 8.1) and may be a useful resource.

Returning to interpersonal issues, participants are asked if they have confidants. Social and emotional support is an important aspect of illness management. The availability of a confidant, whether it be a family member, close friend, clergyman, or therapist, can have an important moderating influence on the stress of debilitating symptoms (see pp. 162–165). CFS support groups and patient newsletters are another source of support that should be introduced and discussed.

Because patients are buffeted by the ongoing intrusions of their illness and its limitations, feelings of emotional and physical stress are often intense and persistent. Relaxation exercises may represent their first exposure to a nondrug technique that can reduce stress, increase their sense of well-being, and improve their sleep (see pp. 140–145). The final 15 minutes of the first group session are devoted to a therapist-guided relaxation procedure. Participants are encouraged to get comfortable in their chairs while lights are dimmed, if possible. The therapist will then deliver relaxation suggestions in a lilting monotone voice using the breathing-focus procedure.

At the end of the calming exercise, participants are asked if they feel more relaxed. If not, what thoughts and feelings interfered with the procedure? (A discussion of relaxation difficulties and possible solutions may be found on p. 141). The breathing-focus technique is assigned for home use, 10 minutes in the morning, 10 minutes in the afternoon, and also at bedtime if they have trouble falling or staying asleep. The technique should be done in a quiet setting before meals.

Sessions 2 and 3

Participants are first asked how often they practiced the previously assigned relaxation exercise and what benefits they received, such as a sense of ease and comfort, improved coping with stress, or better sleep. The therapist encourages continued use of the relaxation exercise in their daily schedules as well as targeted applications of the calming technique to moderate stressful feelings.

As a cognitive-awareness exercise, clients are then asked how much thinking they do about the illness on a daily basis, and what specific thoughts they have. A common stress-related thought involves persistent dwelling on symptoms (e.g., "I'm so sick, I'm so sick"), which produces discouragement and frustration. Other illness-related cognitions include anger-producing thoughts such as "I should be able to do more," "I should be able to control this illness," and "I can't stand this anymore," and self-esteem–related thoughts, including "I'm useless (or weak)." Rational–emotive methods may be used to dispute these stress-inducing beliefs, and coping statements may be generated to reinforce healthy thinking (see pp. 159–161).

The frustrating and unsuccessful attempts by the patient to maintain pre-illness autonomy and functioning may lead to help-seeking behavior. The next therapy issue addresses the patient's ability to request assistance from others when they need it. Each patient is asked how he or she feels about requesting physical help. People with CFS do not like feeling dependent, but they sometimes require others' assistance to do or finish up daily tasks at home or elsewhere. The therapist makes the point that asking for physical assistance may be uncomfortable, but it is neither a disgrace nor a justification to diminish personal worth.

Finally, an imagery exercise may be used as another vehicle to uncover conflicts related to the illness. It is explained to the participants that many of the chronic stressors in their daily life, including the illness, cannot be solved in any immediate or obvious way. The therapist suggests that their ability to cope with chronic stressors can be strengthened. Patients are given a brief relaxation exercise followed by suggestions that they are taking a pleasant walk in the forest where they discover a box (Tubesing & Tubesing, 1983). They enter the box and close it, and describe to themselves the size, color, and texture of the box, and how they feel inside the box. (Prior to this exercise, the therapist should advise claustrophobic patients to avoid the thought of entering the box if it is too stressful. Instead they can imagine another challenge, such as climbing over the box.)

When they exit the box, a personal strategy is developed to make that exit. Brief relaxation is once again given, followed by the participants' drawing a picture of the box with pen and paper. Then they share their experiences about the box image. Did they feel confined, did they feel safe, upset? As homework they are asked to write a dialogue with the box that they drew. The box should represent one of their current ongoing stressors. They begin a dialogue with the box, letting the box speak to them first.

Box: I am (your problem) and here's something I've got to say to
       you:_____ .
You: (*Write your response.*)
Box: (*Let the conversation flow.*)

Their assignment is to write down the dialogue with the box for discussion in the next session. This activity allows clients to better identify their cognitive and emotional reactions to chronic stressors. The concrete image of a box facilitates a dispassionate appraisal of the actual stressor. In addition to this exercise, participants are asked for the next session to list 10 things that make them angry. Anger is a predominant issue in CFS that often arises from the limitations and rejections they have received from others who dismiss the reality of the illness.

Sessions 4 and 5

Patients are asked to read out loud their dialogue with their box, and what they discovered about dealing with that chronic stressor. This exercise offers a new avenue of insight into how clients deal with chronic stressors, and it will allow the therapist to address their specific difficulties in coping with persistent problems.

Next, the anger list is read aloud by each participant. Often, a strong group identification develops with illness-related items on their anger lists. The permission and right to express intense anger in the supportive group milieu provides a healthy emotional release for participants. As anger items are announced and discussed, the therapist and other participants offer support and coping suggestions that can facilitate anger reduction.

To introduce another type of cognitive coping skill, clients are asked if they use affirmations, which are succinct phrases designed to motivate and inspire. Affirmations act as cues to sustain optimism, self-esteem, and direct meaningful activity. Ask clients if they could use a particular affirmation as a coping thought. Affirmations may be in sentence form, such as "I'm entitled to take time for myself" or consist of a single significant word, such as *strength* or *courage*.

Given that the discussion of anger may have emotionally activated participants in a negative way, the remaining 10–15 minutes of the session are devoted to a relaxation technique. Relaxation tapes for home use are also provided. Now that clients are practiced in the techniques of self-relaxation, a prerecorded tape can deepen their experience of calm as well as distract them from body and symptom focusing which may prevent full relaxation. Participants are also directed to compose a list of 10 things that make them laugh to be discussed in the next session.

Session 6

The session begins with a discussion of each client's practical application of coping skills, as acquired in the first five visits, including self-relaxation and cognitive strategies. Did they successfully handle any particular stress since the last session? How did they do it? Illness-related stressors are especially relevant. Then the relaxation tapes provided in Session 5 are reviewed for their efficacy in producing relaxation.

Next, the personal lists of humor items assigned in the previous session are read aloud by all participants. It is prefaced by the therapist's promoting the health-enhancing and stress-reducing value of humor and laughter, based on empirical studies (see p. 147):

> Laughter is a natural tension reducer, a natural pain-reliever; it releases endorphins, which in turn reduces stress. Laughter can even improve physical fitness because it does involve increased heart rate and significant movement of the facial muscles. Finally, laughter entices people to want to be around you.

Participants are polled about how much laughter they express in their daily routine and encouraged to incorporate humor-oriented strategies in ordinary daily activities. A discussion of the humor lists often produces substantial mood elevation during the session. As an assignment for Session 7, clients are instructed to write down their daily activities for the upcoming week. Across the top of a sheet of paper the following headings are listed: Day/Time, Activity or Rest, Fatigue Rating (0–10), Stress Rating (0–10). The purpose of the exercise is to understand how clients divide their daily schedule into work and rest and to chart their stress and fatigue reactions. This information may suggest new ideas for pacing activity, to be discussed in the following session.

Session 7

The 7-day chart of activity, stress, and symptoms is reviewed for each client in order to determine the adequacy of rest periods. Are clients overexerting themselves to exhaustion? Can healthy rest or leisure intervals be incorporated into their daily schedule? The issue of activity pacing (see p. 148) is discussed as a constructive adaptation to the wide and unpredictable symptom fluctuations in CFS. How do clients arrange their daily activities? Are they falling into an overwork–collapse pattern? Or are they more carefully watching their energy levels and allowing rest intervals? Of course, healthy pacing may not be possible if the individual is working full-time, but the ability to balance activity, rest, and leisure is an important behavioral issue for the person with CFS. The therapist and the other group members can suggest behavioral changes for each client to accommodate energy fluctuations. For instance, the therapist may introduce the option of deciding to expend energy on an enjoyable activity, knowing that a setback is risked.

Next, the group is polled about cognitive complaints associated with their illness, including difficulties with short-term memory and sustained concentration. The clinician can ask how they handle these deficits and suggest additional ideas about how to compensate for these difficulties (see pp. 166–168), including minimizing distractions, doing one thing at a time, establishing a routine to reduce confusion, and incorporating written reminders such as wall charts and appointment books for easily forgotten items.

Finally, clients are asked, "Despite the overwhelming negatives of CFS, is there anything positive that has resulted from the illness?" Positive outcomes may include a less frenetic lifestyle, more time for relaxation, or greater appreciation of close interpersonal relationships. As homework for Session 8, participants are directed to compose a list of things they would like to do and could do (despite illness limitations) but are not now doing. Such pleasurable, reinforcing activities can have a substantial mood-elevating, symptom-reducing effect in CFS.

Session 8

To start the group interaction, participants are asked to identify the activities from their prepared lists that they would like to do but are not doing. Each client should be encouraged to plan to carry out a particular activity that they would enjoy very much. The health-producing effects of pleasant mood are then described (see p. 145).

Finally, participants are asked how they benefited from the group sessions. How do they feel now as compared with the initial visit? Are they acting or behaving any differently? Generally, their ability to relax and reduce stress will have improved. They may also experience fewer bouts of sad or depressed moods. New lifestyle adjustments will have allowed them to enjoy leisure time and be more selective about their activities. For some participants, increased physical or mental activity may be reported. These questions will help participants appreciate the gains that they have made and may provoke positive suggestions about illness management on a variety of topics. This discussion will end the group session on a positive note. At the end of the sessions, clients complete Time 2 questionnaire assessments, using the measures of the initial assessment. This termination assessment is useful to confirm and quantify the emotional and behavioral changes that have occurred.

Service Needs and
Community Intervention

12

n this chapter, we examine the service needs of CFS patients and describe the community interventions that have been proven effective with this population. The treating psychotherapist may find this information useful in helping the CFS patient secure community-based practical and emotional support as well as flexible part-time employment.

Individuals with CFS are overwhelmingly tired, sometimes finding even brief conversations to be energy draining. In an effort to conserve energy, particularly during the worst phases of the illness, many individuals with CFS isolate themselves from friends, family, and work. Given the difficulties of maintaining employment, many CFS-affected individuals have limited financial resources, and thus, may be forced to seek less-than-desirable housing. It is not surprising that many CFS-affected people, feeling ill and isolated with limited means, are confronted with an escalating spiral of emotional and physical stressors. Often, a 1-hour-a-month self-help group is all that is available to cope with the illness. Antoni et al. (1994) suggested that those CFS patients who engage in self-blame and avoid discussions about physical limitations may experience a sense of social isolation that is distressing and, without the buffering effects of social support, they might negatively amplify how much their lives have been compromised by their fatigue.

A qualitative study by N. C. Ware and Kleinman (1992) obtained CFS patients' detailed narrative accounts of their illness. CFS sufferers described themselves as living overcommitted and overextended lives, with a tendency to place the interests of others before their own. The data suggested that those who develop this illness may have adopted a social norm that features exhaustion as a way of life. A large percentage of the sample attributed their illness partially or wholly to stress. Those individuals who reported at follow-up that their physical condition had improved had made positive, stress-reducing changes in their personal lives (e.g., changed jobs, were reunited with their families). Similarly, Ray, Jefferies, and Weir (1995b) found that positive life events may contribute to the process of recovery in CFS.

Predictors of improvements, also identified in an 18-month follow-up investigation of 246 patients with CFS (Vercoulen, Swanink, Fennis, et al., 1996), included a subjective sense of control over symptoms, lowered fatigue, shorter duration of complaints, and a relative absence of physical attribution as the cause of their CFS. Only 3% of these patients reported complete recovery, whereas 17% reported improvement. It is possible that these discouraging follow-up statistics are due in part to the isolation arising from the severity of the syndrome and the lack of effective supports available in the community to help people with CFS recover. In addition, the most dramatic changes in health status might occur in those who are able to make constructive changes in their social situations, as was found in the N. C. Ware and Kleinman (1992) study.

Assessment of Service Needs

Comprehensive approaches to treatment should address a variety of care needs. The service needs of the individual with CFS have been discussed by clinicians and scholars. For example, government support for appropriate medical treatment has been cited as a high-priority need for individuals with CFS (D. S. Bell, 1991; Collinge, 1993). In addition, people with CFS may benefit from an advocacy program to educate the general public and the medical community about the problems and difficulties associated with CFS.

Practical help and support may also be important: Some CFS patients may require assistance from others in order to complete daily living tasks. Cooperative living arrangements with healthy individuals who do daily, mundane activities may be necessary for people with CFS because illness-related weakness might prevent them from accomplishing necessary chores (Shafran, 1991). Finally, a sense of

Mean Score and Standard Deviation on Rating Scales Addressing
Rehabilitation Needs

Service	M	SD
Create a telephone "hotline" for PWCs to call for recovery advice and assistance	4.73	0.65
Create an advocacy system for PWCs during their recovery	4.60	0.70
Establish a system of volunteer caregivers for PWCs	4.57	0.81
Establish regular self-help meetings for PWCs with informational speakers	4.53	0.85
Establish regular self-help meetings for PWCs to provide emotional support	4.18	1.10
Create a training center for PWCs to learn recovery strategies and methods	4.05	1.15
Offer "health retreats" for PWCs	3.78	1.27
Provide drop-in social settings for PWCs	3.49	1.30
Screen all well persons living in a home with PWCs	3.45	1.36
Create a referral service to find shared living space for PWCs	3.35	1.38
Create a mixed-home with student caregivers and PWCs; democratically operated	3.25	1.38
Create a democratic, self-governed home for only PWCs;	2.93	1.38
create a mixed-home with separate social space for PWCs	2.85	1.22
Provide limited-duration living space for PWCs with healthy families	2.85	1.34

Note: PWCs = Persons with CFS; *N* = 984 PWCs.

community social support may prevent isolation, depression, and preoccupation with the illness among CFS patients (Blakely et al., 1991; Ray et al., 1993). A key question concerns the highest priority needs, especially from the perspective of the patient with CFS.

To assess more effectively the needs of people with CFS, Jason, Ferrari, Taylor, Slavich, and Stenzel (1996) analyzed a brief questionnaire that assessed the participants' use of and preference for a variety of services. The inventory consisted of fourteen 5-point (1 = *undesirable*; 5 = *extremely desirable*) rating scales. Respondents indicated their preference for each of the 14 hypothetical rehabilitation services that might assist in their recovery from chronic illness. Table 12.1 presents the mean scores and standard deviations for each of the items. As noted in the table, mean scores across items ranged from about 3 to 5.

A principal components factor analysis, performed on the set of 14 scaled items yielded a three-factor solution, with 53.9% of the common variance explained. Factor 1 contained *housing services*, Factor 2 indicated *self-help and social support services*, and Factor 3 consisted of *general advocacy services*. General advocacy services were preferred to a significantly greater extent than self-help and social support services and housing services.

It is not surprising that the highest-rated factor was advocacy services, given the discrimination and negative attitudes that people with this disorder often encounter. Preferred advocacy efforts included (a) a telephone hotline service to provide immediate advice and assistance on illness-related issues, (b) an advocacy worker to secure financial resources and legitimize the service needs of individuals with CFS, and (c) a volunteer caregiver system to offer assistance with daily chores and errands. Respondents with CFS also made a strong plea for education within the medical field, the government, and the general public to increase the awareness of CFS as a genuine disease entity. In turn, such recognition could improve the quality of medical care, enhance financial resources, and increase services offered for individuals with CFS.

The second-highest priority items were self-help groups providing emotional support and current treatment information. This result is consistent with other studies (e.g., Antoni et al., 1994; Blakely et al., 1991) indicating that individuals with CFS may benefit from continued social and emotional support to cope effectively with their illness.

One way to provide these illness-related services would involve the development of a center for patient advocacy and support services. A facility of this type could act as an ombudsman to secure comprehensive services and treatment as a vehicle to recovery. Clearly, these findings suggest that many resources may be necessary to help individuals who have chronic fatigue syndrome.

Buddy–Mentor Intervention

An example of a new community service program for people with CFS involves a buddy–mentor system. Although this type of helping system is common for people with other chronic illnesses (e.g., AIDS), few of these programs have been described in the CFS literature. Investigators at DePaul University devised and evaluated a buddy–mentor system for people with CFS (Schlaes & Jason, 1996). The role of the buddy was to provide emotional support, social companionship, and instrumental support. The buddy was a person in the community who agreed to spend 1 hour a week conducting home visits with a CFS-affected individual. Buddies were matched with the participants based on needs and interests assessments completed by the participants and buddies. Mentors were individuals with CFS who were willing and able to engage in 2 hours of phone contact each month with the participants to provide informational and emotional support.

Participants with CFS who received the buddy–mentor intervention experienced significant declines in fatigue severity, whereas the no-intervention control group experienced significant increases in fatigue severity. Those who received the intervention also reported improvements in positive thinking (Life Orientation Test), whereas the control group experienced decreased levels of positive thinking that approached statistical significance. There were no significant differences in outcome between the experimental and control groups on measures of depression, psychological distress, perceived stress, coping strategies, or perceived social support.

Why was fatigue significantly decreased for the intervention group? One possible reason is that the buddy–mentor program provided resources for people with CFS that may have allowed more time for needed rest. Participants received 1 hour per week of physical support during which the buddy would complete activities such as grocery shopping or housework. Even with this relatively small activity reduction, participants experienced declines in fatigue. This result occurred without declines in measures of psychological functioning, social support, and coping. It is possible that people with CFS experienced improvements in fatigue because they were provided services that lessened their physical strain and exertion.

Not only do people with CFS benefit from having helpers, but volunteers can and do benefit from the volunteer experience as well. Ferrari and Jason (1997) found that caregivers to people with CFS consistently reported more satisfaction than stress from caregiving. This demonstrates that caregiving, in and of itself, can be a fulfilling experience that satisfies personal and emotional needs for the caregiver. By working directly with CFS-affected people, volunteers can learn a great deal about the lives of people with disabilities and the obstacles they need to overcome on a daily basis.

Work Rehabilitation

Many people with CFS are too tired to work. Loss of work can be a devastating and demoralizing experience (Jason, Kolak, et al., 1998). Those affected with CFS often believe that there is little hope of finding employment, particularly employment with a flexible schedule that could accommodate unpredictable and widely fluctuating energy levels. Flexibility at the work site is a key requirement for people with

CFS in search of part-time employment. Furthermore, individuals with CFS are often chemically sensitive and may require jobs that are relatively chemical-free. For example, a freshly painted office or newly installed carpet might trigger a severe symptomatic reaction in some people with CFS.

People diagnosed with CFS are eligible for services provided by the 1992 Amendments to the Rehabilitation Act of 1973. This Act defines the term *individual with a disability* as any individual who has a physical or mental impairment that (a) is a substantial impediment to employment and (b) can benefit in terms of an employment outcome from vocational rehabilitation services. Clearly, people who are disabled by CFS are eligible for services provided by this Act. The 1992 Amendments to the Rehabilitation Act of 1973 specifies the following:

> Individuals with disabilities, including individuals with the most severe disabilities, are generally presumed to be capable of engaging in gainful employment; individuals with disabilities must be provided opportunities to obtain gainful employment in integrated settings; individuals must be active participants in their own rehabilitation programs, including making meaningful and informed choices about the selection of their vocational goals, objectives, and services; families and natural supports can play an important role in the success of an individual's vocational rehabilitation program; qualified rehabilitation personnel can facilitate the employment goals of the individual with a disability.

Community agencies are needed to provide programs that evaluate job-readiness skills to help formerly successful people with CFS return to gainful employment. As some of the surveys previously cited indicate, many people with CFS will benefit from a return to (at least part-time) employment, particularly because their personal identity and self-worth have been associated with work.

To enable people with CFS to return to work, two important factors have to be evaluated: (a) Is the individual employable? (b) Is the individual placeable? Geist and Calzaretta (1982) defined *employability* as the capacity of the individual to function in a particular occupation or work situation. Both general employability and specific employability must be evaluated. The following factors must be considered in evaluating specific employability: general concentration, general attention, ability to attend to the task at hand, ability to attend to detail, stress tolerance, fatigability, emotional and physical endurance, and general work stamina. Geist and Calzaretta (1982) defined *placeability* as the capacity of the individual, with his/her own strengths and weaknesses, to become employed. An individual's placeability varies from time to time depending on the state of the job market and the quality of the individual's preparation for job placement activities. Placeability is often affected by behaviors that have little or nothing to do with the individual's qualifications or knowledge of the job (e.g., punctuality, absenteeism, and interpersonal interactions). For the CFS individual, issues such as the need for breaks and rest may affect his or her placeability.

Heiman (1994) surveyed a sample of people with CFS and found that the median income loss per year was $13,000. In addition, the respondents strongly endorsed the following types of work-related intervention: professional assistance in negotiating with their employees for accommodation, reduction of stress factors at work, assistance with career change, change in working conditions, job sharing, doing some work at home, and flexible hours.

It would be desirable to design and evaluate a project for reemployment based on individually written rehabilitation plans that incorporate medical, psychological, social, and vocational data. Such programs could offer services such as counseling on CFS-affected personal relationships, stress and relaxation procedures, coping with memory and concentration difficulties, job-readiness skill attainment, job placement counseling, and information on proper diet. It would be useful to create many such demonstration projects for individuals confronted with this debilitating condition.

Regrettably, there are few job-related programs for people with CFS. Most agencies are not sure how to develop supportive programs for people with severe energy problems. Because individuals with this syndrome often look healthy when they come into service agencies seeking job counseling or other services, the service providers often do not understand that CFS-affected people might have only a few functional hours each week to give to an employer. Full-time employment is not physically possible for many people with this syndrome. Rather, the person with CFS would benefit from support and encouragement, job assessment, and part-time job opportunities with gradually increasing working hours as endurance and energy improve.

Employment Opportunities

In order to address these employment issues more effectively, a member of the DePaul University research team formed a committee with a group of people with CFS to develop a job bank (Jason, Kolak, et al., 1998). A well-known disability lawyer was invited to attend one of the meetings and share his knowledge in this area. The committee decided to create a job bank listing part-time jobs that might be appropriate for people with CFS. For instance, some home-based employment opportunities, such as multilevel marketing, proofreading, home office computing, and pet-sitting, might allow people with CFS to set their own work schedules. The DePaul researcher and six people with CFS began meeting on a monthly basis to locate and review a variety of part-time jobs. Once a potential part-time job was located, it was placed into the job bank.

The part-time job committee also gave members a chance to receive emotional support and encouragement with the goal of rejoining the workforce, even on a part-time basis. (In general, the support groups allow participants to reduce their sense of isolation, develop a sense of confidence, and have a forum to discuss common problems [Maton, 1989].) In addition to creating a job directory, members have used some of the suggested job leads in their pursuit of part-time work. The job directory continues to be updated and is available to all members of the Chicago Chronic Fatigue Syndrome Association.

On-Line Support

Many people with disabilities are turning to on-line support chat rooms. The possibility of giving and receiving support without having to leave one's home has many benefits, particularly for people with mobility problems. This new system for developing connections between people who have had similar experiences provides a unique, low-cost form of service delivery for people with (and without) disabilities.

We have also found that, within America Online, there is a subdirectory of chat rooms designed specifically for support, the Personal Empowerment Network (PEN). Each chat room has a designated leader or "facilitator" for the group that is chosen from among the participants. Chat rooms are often small, which limits the number of participants. Such a forum might provide a source of comfort for people with CFS where they can be understood and have the opportunity to exchange knowledge and experiences with others.

Chat rooms represent a new type of community for people with CFS. In these rooms, a wide range of individuals participate, from those who have recently been diagnosed with CFS to those who have been ill for many years. There are members who are relatively recovered and those who are extremely disabled. In addition, these discussions are open to individuals without CFS. Thus, others can learn about the daily issues and problems expressed by people with CFS, and this knowledge can help reduce negative stereotypes.

Other University–Self-Help Group Collaborations

Volunteers from DePaul University have also assisted the Chicago Chronic Fatigue Syndrome Association in other capacities. For example, one research assistant helped the CFS group leader create a directory of resources for people with CFS. This resource directory has now become an important asset to the organization, and its sales generate income for the self-help association. Members of our research team have also helped the CFS group leader to assemble and mail the association's newsletter and to reorganize their filing system. The assistance of healthy volunteers in these types of activities has been well received by the members of the CFS self-help group, and it has increased their commitment to our collaborative relationship.

Through work with the various University–CFS self-help group collaborative committees, we have discovered that support groups can help people with CFS overcome some of the difficulties they face. It is our hope that these committees will one day become part of a center to serve people with CFS and others with disabilities.

Conclusion

In this chapter, the concept of professionally initiated community interventions has been applied to the problems and needs of people with CFS. Kelly (1985, 1987) posited that ecological principles should be used by professionals who maintain long-term collaborative relationships with persons and settings. By involving participants actively in the planning of interventions, the recipients of the programs receive support, learn to identify resources, and become better problem-solvers. Change efforts that are not well integrated into the target population and their environment are unlikely to produce effects that will last. On the other hand, interventions that have been generated from collaboratively defined, produced, and implemented change efforts are most apt to endure. These principles are especially relevant to people with CFS, who are a chronically ill population with their own special needs.

Case Definitions of CFS

A

Five definitions of CFS have been proposed, three from the United States (Holmes, Kaplan, Gantz, et al., 1988; Fukuda et al., 1994; Schluederberg et al., 1992), one from Great Britain (Sharpe et al., 1991), and the last one from Australia (Lloyd et al., 1990).

U.S. CASE DEFINITIONS

Initial Definition

The original Holmes, Kaplan, Gantz, et al. (1988) criteria are as follows: A case of CFS must fulfill major criteria 1 and 2, plus the following minor criteria: 6 or more of the 11 symptom criteria and 2 or more of the 3 physical criteria; or 8 or more of 11 symptom criteria. In a letter to the *Annals of Internal Medicine*, several of the authors of this definition suggested that CFS could be diagnosed in the presence of a mood disorder if it occurred after the onset of chronic fatigue (Holmes, Kaplan, Schonberger, et al., 1988). Holmes (1991) stated that this definition is intentionally restrictive, and by emphasizing specificity over sensitivity, noncases will be excluded at the expense of excluding some cases.

Major Criteria

1. New onset of persistent or relapsing, debilitating fatigue or easy fatigability in a person who has no previous history of similar symptoms, that does not resolve with bedrest, and that is severe enough to reduce or impair average daily

activity below 50% of the patient's premorbid activity level for a period of at least 6 months.

2. Other clinical conditions that may produce similar symptoms must be excluded by thorough evaluation (history, physical examination, and appropriate laboratory findings).

Minor Criteria

Symptoms must have begun at or after the time of onset of increased fatigability, and must have persisted or recurred over a period of at least 6 months. Symptoms include the following:

1. Mild fever or chills: oral temperature 37.5 C–38.6 C
2. Sore throat
3. Painful lymph nodes (anterior or posterior cervical or axillary)
4. Unexplained generalized muscle weakness
5. Muscle discomfort or myalgia
6. Prolonged (24 hours or greater) generalized fatigue after levels of exercise that would have been easily tolerated in the patient's premorbid state
7. Generalized headaches (different from type patient may have had in premorbid state)
8. Migratory arthralgia (without joint swelling or redness)
9. Neuropsychiatric complaints (one or more of the following: photophobia, scotomata, forgetfulness, excessive irritability, confusion, difficulty in thinking or concentrating, depression)
10. Sleep disturbance (hypersomnia or insomnia)
11. Description of main symptom complex as initially developing over a few hours to a few days

Physical Criteria

Physical criteria must be documented by a physician on at least two occasions, at least one month apart, and include the following:

1. Low-grade fever: oral temperature of 37.6 C–38.6 C or rectal temperature of 37.8 C–38.8 C
2. Nonexudative pharyngitis
3. Palpable or tender anterior posterior cervical or axillary lymph nodes, (lymph nodes greater than 2 cm in diameter suggest other causes; further evaluation is warranted)

The preceding definition has been used by the Centers for Disease Control (CDC). They used a four-part system for classifying CFS-afflicted people in their prevalence study (Gunn et al., 1993). For Group 1, individuals were diagnosed as meeting the working case definition of CFS (patients with psychiatric illnesses following onset of CFS were included). For Group 2, individuals had unexplained fatigue, but their symptom number or severity did not fully meet the case definition. For Group 3, individuals had evidence of a known medical illness that could cause the fatigue. For Group 4, people had a psychological condition that was diagnosed prior to the onset of fatigue.

Physicians using the CDC definition have made several changes in the Holmes, Kaplan, Gantz, et al. (1988) criteria for diagnosing CFS. For example, major criterion 1 has been defined in the following way: The average daily activity level or energy level below 50% of the patient's premorbid state for a period of at least 6 months (Gunn et al., 1993). In addition, four psychiatric disorders (somatization, depression, panic disorder, and generalized anxiety disorder) are not exclusionary, if they occurred after the onset of CFS. In a discussion found in Gunn et al. (1993), Dr. Abbey stated that there has been a shift in the thinking of the Physician Review Committee group, so that when a preceding psychiatric history was a clearly isolated incident that could not be implicated in the subsequent CFS, the patient would be placed in Group 1 rather than Group 4. Dr. Abbey also mentioned that "it is clear to my psychiatrist's eye that they [some patients] do not have CFS, but rather primary psychiatric disorder which has been misdiagnosed" (p. 97), and yet because of the decision tree being used, some of these patients qualify for Group 1 and get counted as CDC-defined CFS with concurrent psychopathology.

Second Definition

A second definition of CFS is a modified version of the Holmes, Kaplan, Gantz, et al. (1988) criteria, using rules developed at the 1991 National Institute of Allergy and Infectious Disease/National Institute of Mental Health workshop on CFS (as reported in Schluederberg et al., 1992), and includes the following recommendations:

1. *Exclusions from the case definition*: psychiatric disorder—psychoses (psychotic depression, bipolar disorder, schizophrenia, etc.); substance abuse; postinfectious fatigue in which a definite etiology has been established and the clinical picture is compatible with ongoing, active infection, (e.g., chronic hepatitis B with active liver disease, HIV infection, Lyme disease [inadequately treated]).

2. *Inclusions in the case definition*: fibromyalgia (identified by established criteria/tender point exam; stratify in studies);

postinfectious fatigues (stratify in studies)—Lyme disease with persistent fatigue after appropriate antibiotic therapy; brucellosis with persistent fatigue after appropriate antibiotic therapy; a chronic debilitating fatigue that follows well-documented cases of acute infectious mononucleosis, acute CMV (cytomegalovirus) infection, and acute adequately-treated toxoplasmosis; depression (nonpsychotic)—depression (stratify in studies), concurrent, 1 month postonset or 6 months or more before onset (stratify in studies); other disorder—panic disorder (with or without agoraphobia), generalized anxiety disorder, and somatoform disorder (stratify in studies).

3. *Description of onset and response to therapy*: Timing of onset of disorder (e.g., one discrete and self-limited episode well before the onset of chronic fatigue; chronic and recurring episodes well before the onset of chronic fatigue; active at the time of onset of chronic fatigue; clearly beginning after the onset of chronic fatigue). Also classify by response to therapy (Does the psychiatric disorder improve, and does the chronic fatigue and associated somatic symptoms improve?).

Current Definition

The third definition of CFS, which is now used by investigators in the United States, was created by Fukuda et al. (1994). They defined prolonged fatigue as 1 month or more, and chronic fatigue is defined as self-reported persistent or relapsing fatigue for 6 or more consecutive months.

The following four steps should be included in the assessment:

1. A thorough history should be conducted concerning the medical and psychosocial circumstances at the onset of the fatigue. In addition, information should be gathered on current use of prescriptions, over-the-counter drugs, or food supplements.
2. A mental status exam should give attention to current anxiety, self-destructive thoughts, or psychomotor retardation. If there is evidence of a psychiatric or neurological disorder, there should be an appropriate psychiatric, psychological, or neurological evaluation.
3. A physical exam should be conducted.
4. Necessary laboratory tests should be conducted.

Conditions that exclude chronic fatigue are the following:

1. An active medical condition that explains chronic fatigue (e.g., untreated hypothyroidism, sleep apnea, medication side effects)
2. A previously diagnosed medical disorder whose resolution has not been documented beyond reasonable clinical doubt and whose continued activity may explain the chronic fatiguing illness (e.g., unresolved cases of hepatitis B or C)
3. Past or current major depression with melancholic or psychotic features, delusional disorders, bipolar affective disorder, schizophrenia, anorexia nervosa, or bulimia
4. Alcohol or substance abuse within 2 years before the onset of CFS or at anytime afterward
5. Severe obesity (body mass index greater than or equal to 45)

The following are not excluded:

1. Conditions that are defined by symptoms that cannot be confirmed by diagnostic laboratory tests (e.g., fibromyalgia, anxiety disorders, multiple chemical disorder, somatoform disorders, nonpsychotic or nonmelancholic depression, neurasthenia)
2. Conditions under specific treatment sufficient to alleviate all symptoms related to that condition, for example, treated and controlled hypothyroidism
3. Any disease such as Lyme disease or syphilis that was treated with definitive therapy before the onset of chronic symptomatic sequelae
4. Any unexplained physical examination finding or laboratory abnormality that is insufficient to strongly suggest the existence of an exclusionary condition.

After the preceding steps have been completed, a case is then defined as follows: (a) CFS is clinically evaluated, unexplained, persistent or relapsing chronic fatigue that is of new or definite onset (i.e., not lifelong); the fatigue is not the result of ongoing exertion, is not substantially alleviated by rest, and results in substantial reductions in previous levels of occupational, educational, social, or personal activities. (b) There must be concurrent occurrence of four or more of the following symptoms, and all must be persistent or recurrent during 6 or more months of the illness and not predate the fatigue:

1. Self-reported persistent or recurrent impairment in short-term memory or concentration severe enough to cause substantial reductions in previous levels of occupational, educational, social, or personal activities
2. Sore throat
3. Tender cervical or axillary lymph nodes
4. Muscle pain
5. Multiple joint pain without joint swelling or redness
6. Headaches of a new type, pattern, or severity
7. Unrefreshing sleep
8. Postexertional malaise lasting more than 24 hours

BRITISH CASE DEFINITION

A fourth set of criteria comprises the British definition of CFS, proposed by Sharpe et al. (1991). To fulfill their criteria, patients must have met the following guidelines for CFS:

1. A syndrome characterized by fatigue as the principal symptom
2. A syndrome of definite onset that is not lifelong
3. Fatigue that is severe, disabling, and affects physical and mental functioning
4. Presence of the symptom of fatigue for a minimum of six months during which time it was present for more than 50% of the time
5. Possible presence of other symptoms, particularly myalgia, mood, and sleep disturbance
6. Exclusion of certain patients from the definition as follows:
   a. Patients with established medical conditions known to produce chronic fatigue (e.g., severe anemia), who should be excluded whether the medical condition is diagnosed at presentation or only subsequently. All patients should have a history and physical examination performed by a competent physician.
   b. Patients with a current diagnosis of schizophrenia, bipolar affective disorder, substance abuse, eating disorder, or proven organic brain disease. Other psychiatric disorders (including depressive illness, anxiety disorders, and hyperventilation syndrome) are not necessarily reasons for exclusion.

In addition, postinfectious fatigue syndrome (PIFS) is a subtype of CFS that either follows an infection or is associated with a current infection (although whether such associated infection is of etiological significance is a topic for research). To meet research criteria for PIFS, patients (a) must fulfill major criteria for CFS as defined above and (b) should also fulfill the following additional criteria:

1. There is definite evidence of infection at onset or presentation (a patient's self-report is unlikely to be sufficiently reliable).
2. The syndrome is present for at least 6 months after onset of infection.
3. The infection has been corroborated by laboratory evidence.

The British definition also provides specific definitions of the terms used above. *Fatigue* is a discrete subjective sensation, and features of fatigue commonly reported are mental and physical aspects. Mental fatigue is characterized by lack of motivation and alertness. Physical fatigue is felt as lack of energy or strength and is often felt in the muscles. The fatigue must be complained of, it must significantly affect the person's functioning, it should be disproportionate to exertion, it should represent a clear change from a previous state, and it must be persistent, or if intermittent, should be present more than 50% of the time.

According to the British definition, *disability* refers to a restriction or lack of ability to perform an activity in the manner or within the range considered normal for a human being in areas of occupational, social, and leisure activities. There should be a definite and persistent change from a previous level of functioning.

Finally, the British definition defines *myalgia* as symptoms of pain or aching felt in the muscles. Myalgia should be complained of, be disproportionate to exertion, be a change from a previous state, and should be persistent or recurrent. *Mood disturbances* include depressed mood, anhedonia (loss of interest and loss of pleasure), anxious mood, emotional lability, and irritability. It should be determined whether the patient's disorder is sufficient to meet operational diagnostic criteria for major depressive disorder, generalized anxiety disorder, or panic disorder. These *mood disorders* should be complained of, should represent a significant change from a previous state, and should be relatively persistent or recurrent. Finally, *sleep disturbances* refer to a subjective report of a change in the duration or quality of sleep. They include hypersomnia (increased sleep) or insomnia (reduced sleep). These sleep disturbances should be complained of, should not be simply a response to external disturbances, should be a change from a previous state, and should be persistent.

AUSTRALIAN CASE DEFINITION

There have been several proposed Australian CFS definitions. We will review the definition used in the Lloyd et al. (1990) epidemiological study. To fulfill the criteria, patients have to have the following symptoms:

1. Chronic persisting or relapsing fatigue of a generalized nature, exacerbated by minor exercise or causing significant disruption of usual daily activities, and present for greater than 6 months
2. Neuropsychiatric dysfunction, including impairment of concentration evidenced by difficulty in completing mental tasks that were easily accomplished before the onset of the syndrome; new onset of short-term memory impairment
3. No alternative diagnosis reached by history, physical examination, or investigations over a 6-month period

In order to fulfill criterion 1, the patient must endorse at least one of the three following items relating to fatigue with a score of 1 ("excessive muscle fatigue with minor activity," "prolonged feeling of fatigue after physical activity [lasting hours or days]"), with a score of 2 ("moderate or frequent symptoms during the last month causing major disruption to your usual daily activities") or with a score of 3 ("severe or very frequent symptoms during the last month making you unable to perform your usual daily activities"). In order to fulfill criterion 2, a patient must have a score of 2 or 3 (same as descriptors above) on at least one of two questions relating to neuropsychiatric dysfunction ("loss of concentrating ability" and "memory loss").

CONCLUSION

None of the current definitions have been empirically derived or prospectively contrasted with one another. Komaroff and Geiger (1989) compared patients who met the CDC case definition with those who did not and found that the CDC criteria did not identify a subgroup of patients more likely to have objective evidence of disease. They concluded that restricting studies to those patients that fully meet the CDC criteria may be unwise. Katon et al. (1991) also found that patients with CFS were indistinguishable from those with chronic fatigue not meeting the CDC criteria. One study that has compared definitions found similar laboratory abnormalities with the CDC, British, and Australian case definitions (Bates et al., 1992). In diagnosing 808 patients (Bates et al., 1992), it was found that 44% were classified with CFS using the CDC criteria, 62% were classified with CFS using the British criteria, and 82% were classified with CFS using the Australian definition.

Appendix

Medical Assessment of CFS

During the physician visit, a structured instrument, such as the CFS questionnaire (developed by Komaroff and Buchwald, 1991), should be administered. This instrument identifies the presenting signs, symptoms, and medical history of the patient in order to rule out other disorders. It also assesses fatigue severity, CFS-related social role impairment, psychosocial stressors, job satisfaction, toxic exposures prior to CFS onset, presence of CFS in other social network members, and family medical history. Because sleep disturbances are often reported by patients with CFS, the Sleep Disturbance Questionnaire (validated by studies in a sleep laboratory; D. Buchwald, R. Pascualy, C. Bombardier, & P. Kith, personal communication, September 3, 1992), can be used to identify patients with sleep disturbances. In some patients studied by Krupp et al. (1991), a sleep disorder and psychiatric condition coexisted to produce a symptom complex resembling CFS. Important medical information should also be gathered to determine other possible medical causes of chronic fatigue, such as exposure histories to tuberculosis, AIDS, and non-AIDS sexually transmitted diseases, and prescribed and illicit drug use. For women, results of recent Pap smears and mammograms need to be obtained. A history of all symptoms related to CFS should also be collected.

The laboratory tests to be included in the battery should be the minimum necessary to rule out other illnesses (Schluederberg et al., 1992), including a chemistry screen (which assesses liver, renal, and thyroid functioning), complete blood count with differential and platelet count, erythrocyte sedimentation rate, arthritic profile (which includes rheumatoid factor and antinuclear antibody), hepatitis B, HIV screen, and urinalysis. A tuberculin skin test should also be performed.

Finally, an anterior–posterior and lateral chest x-ray should be obtained if one has not been obtained within 8 months of the study.

A physician should conduct a detailed medical examination to detect evidence of diffuse adenopathy, hepatosplenomegaly, synovitis, neuropathy, myopathy, or cardiac or pulmonary dysfunction. This evaluation represents a critical part of an assessment because, as noted by Armon and Kurland (1991), in clinical practice it is common for chronically fatigued persons to report that they have a fever or swollen glands or lymph nodes when these are not found during medical examinations. Komaroff and Buchwald (1991) state that unusual or abnormal findings on physical examination are found on 10–50% of CFS patients. An 18-tender-point examination should be used to test for fibromyalgia (Goodnick & Sandoval, 1993). Subsequent workup may necessitate an electrocardiogram, immunoglobulin levels, and serum cortisol determinations, among other tests. Other laboratory studies (e.g., sleep studies) might need to be ordered if deemed necessary.

A variety of medical problems may be encountered in chronic fatigue samples. Manu, Lane, and Matthews (1992a) examined 327 patients with chronic fatigue and found 1% had obstructive sleep apnea, .7% temporal lobe epilepsy, .7% polymyalgia rheumatica, .7% bronchial asthma, .3% hypopituitarism, .3% hypothyroidism, .3% systemic lupus erythematosus (SLE), and 1.2% chronic infections (e.g., Lyme disease, viral hepatitis). There were common minor laboratory abnormalities (anemia, atypical lymphocytosis, elevations of the erythrocyte sedimentation rate, hypophosphatemia, decreased serum iron and total iron binding capacity, and microscopic hematuria), but these produced diagnostic information relevant to the fatigue in fewer than 5% of patients.

The list that follows of medical exclusionary diseases provides only a rough guide for excluding patients from a CFS diagnosis (K. Fukuda, personal communication, Jan. 15, 1993). For example, a chronic fatigue patient who has been previously diagnosed with hypothyroidism and successfully treated would have hypothyroidism excluded as a reason for current, ongoing fatigue. The key issue is for each patient to have a careful medical workup in order to determine if a particular disease is responsible for the fatigue. As is evident, there are multiple causes of fatigue (Podell, 1987). CFS symptoms overlap with many well-recognized illnesses (e.g., Lyme borreliosis, mild SLE, and early or mild MS) and other less common diseases (e.g., Sjogrens syndrome) that might represent frequently overlooked subsets of chronic fatigue patients who have identifiable medical conditions and therefore would be excluded from a diagnosis of CFS (Calabrese, Davis, & Wilke, 1992).

- *Endocrine diseases:* hypothyroidism, Addison's disease, diabetes mellitus, Cushing syndrome,
- *Hematologic diseases:* lymphoma, chronic anemia
- *Neuromuscular and neurologic diseases:* MS, myasthenia gravis, obstructive sleep syndrome
- *Rheumatologic diseases:* polymyalgia rheumatica, polymyositis, Sjogren's syndrome
- *Autoimmune disease*: lupus erythematosus
- *Infections:* HIV, tuberculosis, Lyme disease (inadequately treated; fatigue following properly treated early Lyme disease and brucellosis is not excluded), hepatitis B virus, hepatitis C virus, endocarditis, (chronic debilitating fatigue that persists following a well-documented case of acute infectious mononucleosis or acute cytomegalovirus are not excluded)
- *Fungal diseases:* histoplasmosis, blastomycosis, coccidioidomycosis
- *Parasitic diseases:* toxoplasmosis (don't include if adequately treated), amebiasis, giardiasis, helminthic infestation
- *Chronic inflammatory diseases:* chronic hepatitis, Wegener granulomatosis, sarcoidosis
- *Other chronic diseases:* renal, hepatic, cardiac, gastrointestinal

CFS Symptom Report Form

Name: _____

Date: _____

SYMPTOM RATING FORM

For the symptoms below, please check those symptoms that predate the fatigue illness. Then check those symptoms that persisted or reoccurred during 6 or more months of the fatigue illness.

In the next two columns, please rate the symptoms on a 100-point scale, with 0 = *no pain or problem* and 100 = *severe pain or problem*. Please rate these symptoms during your worst 6-month period of illness, note approximate dates, and also rate the symptoms for how you are experiencing them today.

Approximate dates for worst period: _____

	Predate illness	6 or more months	Rating during worst period	Rating today
Fatigue	_____	_____	_____	_____
Postexertional malaise lasting more than 24 hr	_____	_____	_____	_____
Sore throat	_____	_____	_____	_____
Tender neck or ancillary lymph nodes	_____	_____	_____	_____
Muscle pain	_____	_____	_____	_____
Multiple joint pain without swelling or redness	_____	_____	_____	_____

	Predate illness	6 or more months	Rating during worst period	Rating today
Headaches of a new type, pattern, or severity	___	___	___	___
Unrefreshing sleep	___	___	___	___
Impairments in short-term memory or concentration	___	___	___	___
Other Somatic Complaints				
Racing heart	___	___	___	___
Chest pain	___	___	___	___
Shortness of breath	___	___	___	___
Upset stomach	___	___	___	___
Abdomen pain	___	___	___	___
Weight change	___	___	___	___
Poor Appetite	___	___	___	___
Frequent nauseated feeling	___	___	___	___
Dizziness	___	___	___	___
Ringing in the ears	___	___	___	___
Sweating hands	___	___	___	___
Night sweats	___	___	___	___
Tense muscles	___	___	___	___
Chilled or shivery	___	___	___	___
Hot or cold spells	___	___	___	___
Feeling like you have a temperature	___	___	___	___
Frequent/recurrent fevers	___	___	___	___
Temperature lower than normal	___	___	___	___
Frequent tingling feeling	___	___	___	___
Paralysis	___	___	___	___
Blurred vision	___	___	___	___
Abnormal sensitivity to light	___	___	___	___
Blind spots	___	___	___	___
Eye pain	___	___	___	___
Rash	___	___	___	___
Allergies	___	___	___	___
Chemical sensitivity	___	___	___	___
Muscle weakness	___	___	___	___
Feel unsteady on feet	___	___	___	___
Need to nap during each day	___	___	___	___
Difficulty falling asleep	___	___	___	___
Difficulty staying asleep	___	___	___	___
Other	___	___	___	___

	Predate illness	6 or more months	Rating during worst period	Rating today
Other Cognitive Difficulties				
Slowness of thought	_____	_____	_____	_____
Absent-mindedness	_____	_____	_____	_____
Confusion/disorientation	_____	_____	_____	_____
Difficulty reasoning things out	_____	_____	_____	_____
Forgetting what you are trying to say	_____	_____	_____	_____
Difficulty finding the right word	_____	_____	_____	_____
Difficulty following things	_____	_____	_____	_____
Difficulty understanding	_____	_____	_____	_____
Slow to react	_____	_____	_____	_____
Poor hand to eye coordination	_____	_____	_____	_____
New trouble with math	_____	_____	_____	_____
Concern with driving	_____	_____	_____	_____
Other	_____	_____	_____	_____
Mood Difficulties				
Anxiety/tension	_____	_____	_____	_____
Easily irritated	_____	_____	_____	_____
Depression	_____	_____	_____	_____
Mood swings	_____	_____	_____	_____
Other	_____	_____	_____	_____

Please rate these questions during your worst period of time and today. Mark an *X* next to the appropriate number.

Social/Recreational Activities

Worst period	Today	
_____	_____	0 = Normal levels, before illness
_____	_____	1 = 90%
_____	_____	2 = 80%
_____	_____	3 = 70%
_____	_____	4 = 60%
_____	_____	5 = Half of your normal level
_____	_____	6 = 40%
_____	_____	7 = 30%
_____	_____	8 = 20%
_____	_____	9 = 10%
_____	_____	10 = Completely curtailed

Work Activities

Worst period	Today	
_____	_____	0 = Full-time, without difficulty
_____	_____	1 = Full-time, with difficulty if physical labor is required
_____	_____	2 = Full-time, with difficulty if performing desk activity or light work
_____	_____	3 = 6–7 hr a day at the office, requires rest periods
_____	_____	4 = 4–5 hr a day at the office, requires rest periods
_____	_____	5 = 3 hr a day at the office, requires rest periods
_____	_____	6 = 1–2 hr a day at the office and 1 hr at home, requires rest periods
_____	_____	7 = Only at home 1–2 hr a day
_____	_____	8 = Only at home, 30 min–1 hr a day
_____	_____	9 = Only at home, 5 min–30 min a day
_____	_____	10 = Not able to work at all

Fatigue-Related Cognitions Scale

D

Name: _____

Date: _____

Below are a series of statements regarding your fatigue. By fatigue we mean a sense of tiredness, lack of energy or total body give-out. Please read each statement and circle the number that indicates your level of agreement or disagreement with the statement.

Please answer these questions as they apply to the past TWO WEEKS.

In the past TWO WEEKS, my average level of fatigue was (*circle one*):

1	2	3	4	5	6	7	8	9	10
very mild fatigue				moderate fatigue				severe fatigue	

	Disagree strongly	Disagree moderately	??	Agree moderately	Agree strongly
1. I think about my fatigue often.	1	2	3	4	5
2. I worry if I will be cured of my fatigue.	1	2	3	4	5
3. My fatigue makes me angry.	1	2	3	4	5
4. I need support from family or friends to cope with my fatigue.	1	2	3	4	5
5. It is awful to feel as fatigued as I do.	1	2	3	4	5
6. I sometimes think I deserve the fatigue I feel.	1	2	3	4	5
7. I can't get rid of my fatigue.	1	2	3	4	5

	Disagree strongly	Disagree moderately	??	Agree moderately	Agree strongly
8. I have no control over my fatigue.	1	2	3	4	5
9. I sometimes think I'm dying because my fatigue symptoms are so severe.	1	2	3	4	5
10. Fatigue is very frustrating for me.	1	2	3	4	5
11. I sometimes have suicidal thoughts due to my fatigue.	1	2	3	4	5
12. My fatigue-related limitations make me feel guilty.	1	2	3	4	5
13. I feel sorry for myself as a fatigue victim.	1	2	3	4	5
14. My fatigue helps me get the attention I feel I deserve.	1	2	3	4	5

A Four-Stage Model of CFS: A Coping Tool

E

A progressive four-stage model of the CFS experience (Fennell, 1995a) provides a framework for patients to understand the changing physical, psychological, social, and vocational consequences of their illness. Clinicians may find this experiential model useful in reassuring their patients about illness-related difficulties.

STAGE 1

During the onset of CFS (Stage 1), which may unfold over many years, patients often utilize denial as a functional coping mechanism. As symptoms become more intrusive and disabling, denial may succumb to an escalating crisis of emotional isolation and bewilderment. Family and friends may or may not be supportive. Vocational functioning may be compromised if illness severity limits performance.

STAGE 2

In Stage 2, the initial relief of obtaining a diagnosis of CFS yields to the disappointment, desperation, and fear about the lack of effective treatments or cure. Patients' self-confidence erodes as routine physical and cognitive tasks are done with increasing difficulty. Personal social networks may become more distant as the persistence of the illness continually frustrates the support network. Patients' impairments may lead to a leave of absence from work and the risk of job loss.

STAGE 3

In this stage, individuals maintain an illness plateau but relapses often occur. Relapses may be triggered by desperate attempts to engage in normal tasks or pursuits. Socially, patients undergo even greater loss as friends and significant others may abandon them, resulting in increased feelings of isolation and stigmatization. Further work reductions or terminations may occur.

STAGE 4

At this stage, patients may continue the illness plateau or experience improved health. Some individuals may endure a "plateaued crisis," that is, those who are bedridden. As patients lose faith in medical interventions, they are more likely to emphasize personal efforts to achieve greater control of their lives. Some patients reassess their values and develop new standards for living, whereas others continue their attempts to sustain the roles they held before CFS began.

If values are redefined, new social connections may be found. Patients may turn to new forms of support, such as educational and support organizations or political activism. Others may apply themselves to spiritual paths. Vocational outcomes are highly varied; patients' work schedules or jobs may be modified or completely abandoned for an entirely different type of work. Those with disability benefits may discover new functional options, paid or voluntary, to create meaning and purpose and "make a difference."

As an educational tool, the four-stage model confirms and clarifies the physical and psychosocial consequences of the illness. With such knowledge, patients receive an important sense of validation and reassurance and may develop an improved ability to cope with illness burdens. The four-stage model should be considered an enlightened and flexible psychosocial conceptualization of CFS that may generate a strong identification among individuals with CFS. Empirical studies of the model have recently begun (P. A. Fennell, personal communication, March 22, 1998).

Social Support Scale

F

Think of the people in your life who are important to you. The questions below refer to feelings that you might have about them and the ways in which they respond to you.

Circle one number for each item to indicate the extent to which each description applies. If you wish, you can make a photocopy of the Social Support Scale and fill it out for each significant helper in your life.

Your answer choices are:
1. Never
2. Almost never
3. Sometimes
4. Quite often
5. Very often
6. Always

1. Can you lean on and turn to them when things are difficult?	1	2	3	4	5	6
2. Can you get a good feeling about yourself from them?	1	2	3	4	5	6
3. Do they put pressure on you to do things?	1	2	3	4	5	6
4. Do they take over your chores when you feel ill?	1	2	3	4	5	6
5. Do they express concern about how you are?	1	2	3	4	5	6

Reproduced with permission of author and publisher from: Ray, C. Positive and negative social support in a chronic illness. *Psychological Reports*, 1992, 71, 977–978. © Psychological Reports 1992.

6. Do they misunderstand the way you think and feel about things?	1	2	3	4	5	6
7. Can you trust them, talk frankly, and share your feelings with them?	1	2	3	4	5	6
8. Can you get practical help from them?	1	2	3	4	5	6
9. Do they argue with you about things?	1	2	3	4	5	6
10. Do you feel that they are there when you need them?	1	2	3	4	5	6
11. Do they press you to say that you're feeling better when you're ill?	1	2	3	4	5	6
12. Do they listen when you want to confide about things that are important to you?	1	2	3	4	5	6
13. Do they express irritation with you?	1	2	3	4	5	6
14. Do they accept you as you are, including your failings as well as your stronger points?	1	2	3	4	5	6
15. Do they help out when things need to be done?	1	2	3	4	5	6
16. Do they show you affection?	1	2	3	4	5	6
17. Do they make helpful suggestions about what you should do?	1	2	3	4	5	6
18. Are they critical of the way you respond to illness?	1	2	3	4	5	6
19. Do they do things that conflict with your own sense of what should be done?	1	2	3	4	5	6
20. Do they give you useful advice when you want it?	1	2	3	4	5	6
21. Do they express frustration with you?	1	2	3	4	5	6
22. Do they treat you with respect?	1	2	3	4	5	6
23. Do they disagree with you about what is best for you to do?	1	2	3	4	5	6

References

Abbey, S. E. (1993). Somatization, illness attribution and the sociocultural psychiatry of chronic fatigue syndrome. In B. R. Bock & J. Whelan (Eds.), *Chronic Fatigue Syndrome* (pp. 238–261). New York: Wiley.

Abbey, S. E., & Garfinkel, P. E. (1991a). Chronic Fatigue Syndrome and depression: Cause, effect, or covariate. *Reviews of Infectious Diseases, 13,* S73–S83.

Abbey, S. E., & Garfinkel, P. E. (1991b). Neurasthenia and chronic fatigue syndrome: The role of culture in the making of a diagnosis. *American Journal of Psychiatry, 148,* 1638–1646.

Abbey, S., Toner, B., Garfinkel, P., Kennedy, S., & Kaplan, A. (1990). Self-report symptoms that predict major depression in patients with prominent physical symptoms. *International Journal of Psychiatry in Medicine, 20,* 247–258.

Abbot, N. C., Spence, V. A., Potts, R. C., Lowe, J. G., Belch, J. J. F., & Beck, J. S. (1996, October). *Immune activation markers and cutaneous DHS responses in CFS patients and close family contacts.* Paper presented at the American Association for Chronic Fatigue Syndrome Research Conference, San Francisco, CA.

Ader, R., & Cohen, N. (1975). Behaviorally conditioned immunosuppression. *Psychosomatic Medicine, 37,* 333–340.

Alisky, J. M., Iczkowski, K. A., & Foti, A. A. (1991). Chronic Fatigue Syndrome [Letter to the editor]. *American Family Physician, 44,* 56, 61.

Allen, A. D., & Tilkian, S. M. (1986). Depression correlated with cellular immunity in systemic immunodeficient Epstein-Barr virus syndrome (SIDES). *Journal of Clinical Psychiatry, 47,* 133–135.

American Psychiatric Association. (1994). *Diagnostic and statistical manual of mental disorders* (4th ed.). Washington, DC: Author.

Anderson, J. S., & Ferrans, C. E. (1997). The quality of life of persons with chronic fatigue syndrome. *Journal of Nervous & Mental Disease, 185,* 359–367.

Antoni, M. H., Brickman, A., Lutgendorf, S., Klimas, N., Imia-Fins, A., Ironson, G., Quillian, R., Jose Miguez, M., van Riel, F., Morgan, R., Patarca, R., & Fletcher, M. A. (1994). Psychosocial correlates of illness burden in chronic fatigue syndrome. *Clinical Infectious Diseases, 18*(Suppl. 1), S73–S78.

Armon, C., & Kurland, L. T. (1991). Chronic Fatigue Syndrome: Issues in the diagnosis and estimation of incidence. *Reviews of Infectious Diseases, 13,* S68–S72.

Aronson, K. R., & Barrett, L. F. (1997, August). *The role of emotional reactivity in somatization.* Paper presented at the annual convention of the American Psychological Association, Chicago, IL.

Ax, S., Gregg, V. H., & Jones, D. (1997). Chronic fatigue syndrome—Sufferers' evaluation of medical support. *Journal of the Society of Medicine, 90,* 250–254.

Azar, B. (1997, January). Poor recall mars research and treatment. *The APA Monitor, 28,* 1, 29.

Bakheit, A. M.O., Behan, P. O., Dinan, T. G., Gray, C. E., & O'Keane, V. (1992). Possible upregulation of hypothalamic 5-hydroxytryptamine receptors in patients with postviral fatigue syndrome. *British Medical Journal, 304,* 1010–1012.

Barofsky, I., & Legro, M. W. (1991). Definition and measurement of fatigue. *Reviews of Infectious Diseases, 13,* 94–97.

Barsky, A. (1996, November). *Validity of bodily symptoms in medical outpatients.* Paper presented at the Science of Self-Report meeting at the National Institutes of Health, Bethesda, MD.

Bartley, S. H., & Chute, E. (1969). *Fatigue and impairment in man.* New York: Johnson Reprints.

Bates, D. W., Buchwald, D., Lee, J., Kornish, J., Doolittle, T., & Komaroff, A. L. (1992). A comparison of case definitions of Chronic Fatigue Syndrome [Abstract]. *Clinical Research, 40,* 234A.

Bates, D. W., Buchwald, D., Lee, J., Kornish, J., Doolittle, T. H., Umali, P., & Komaroff, A. L. (1994). A comparison of case definitions of Chronic Fatigue Syndrome. *Clinical Infectious Diseases, 18*(Suppl.), S11–S13.

Bates, D. W., Schmitt, W., Buchwald, D., Ware, N. C., Lee, J., Thoyer, E., Kornish, R. J., & Komaroff, A. L. (1993). Prevalence of fatigue and Chronic Fatigue Syndrome in a primary care practice. *Archives of Internal Medicine, 153,* 2759–2765.

Beard, G. M. (1869). Neurasthenia, or nervous exhaustion. *Boston Medical and Surgical Journal, 3,* 217–221.

Bearn, J., & Wessely, S. (1994). Neurobiological aspects of chronic fatigue syndrome. *European Journal of Clinical Investigation, 24,* 79–90.

Beck, A. J. (1967). *Depression: Clinical, experimental and theoretical aspects.* New York: Harper & Row.

Beh, H. C. (1997). Effect of noise stress on chronic fatigue syndrome patients. *Journal of Nervous & Mental Disease, 185,* 55–58.

Behan, P. O., Behan, W. M. H., & Horrobin, D. (1990). Effects of high doses of essential fatty acids on the postviral fatigue syndrome. *Acta Neurologica Scandinavia, 82,* 209–216.

Bell, D. S. (1991). *The disease of a thousand names.* Lyndonville, NY: Pollard.

Bell, I. (1996, October). *Multiple chemical sensitivity and clinical ecology.* Paper presented at the research conference of the American Association for Chronic Fatigue Syndrome, San Francisco, CA.

Belza, B. L. (1995). Comparison of self-reported fatigue in rheumatoid arthritis and controls. *Journal of Rheumatology, 22,* 639–643.

Belza, B., Henke, C., Yelin, E., Epstein, W., & Gillis, C. (1993). Correlates of fatigue in older adults with rheumatoid arthritis. *Nursing Research, 42,* 93–99.

Bentall, R. P., Wood, G. C., Marrinan, T., Deans, C., & Edwards, R. H. T. (1993). A brief mental fatigue questionnaire. *British Journal of Clinical Psychology, 32,* 375–379.

Berk, L. S. (1989). Neuroendocrine and stress hormone changes during mirthful laughter. *American Journal of Medical Sciences, 298,* 390–396.

Berkman, L. F. (1995). The role of social relations in health promotion. *Psychosomatic Medicine, 57,* 245–254.

Berne, K. (1992). *Running on empty.* Alameda, CA: Hunter House Publishers.

Bernstein, I. H., Jaremko, M. E., & Hinkley, B. S. (1994). On the utility of the SCL-90-R with low back pain patients. *Spine, 19,* 42–48.

Blakely, A. A., Howard, R. C., Sosich, R. M., Murdoch, J. C., Menkes, D. B., & Spears, G. F. S. (1991). Psychiatric symptoms, personality and ways of coping in chronic fatigue syndrome. *Psychological Medicine, 21,* 347–362.

Blalock, S. J., DeVellis, R. F., Brown, G. K., & Wallston, V. A. (1989). Validity of the Center for Epidemiological Studies Depression Scale in arthritis populations. *Arthritis and Rheumatism, 32,* 991–997.

Blondel-Hill, E., & Shafran, S. D. (1993). Treatment of the chronic fatigue syndrome. A review and practical guide. *Drugs, 46,* 639–651.

Bombardier, C. H., & Buchwald, D. (1995). Outcome and prognosis of patients with chronic fatigue versus chronic fatigue syndrome. *Archives of Internal Medicine, 155,* 2105–2110.

Bombardier, C. H., & Buchwald, D. (1996). Chronic fatigue, chronic fatigue syndrome, and fibromyalgia. Disability and health-care use. *Medical Care, 34,* 924–930.

Bonner, D., Ron, M., Chalder, T., Butler, S. & Wessely, S. (1994). Chronic fatigue syndrome: A follow-up study. *Journal of Neurology, Neurosurgery & Psychiatry, 57,* 617–621.

Bonynge, R. R. (1993). Unidimensionality of SCL-90-R scales in adult and adolescent crisis samples. *Journal of Clinical Psychology, 49,* 212–215.

Bou-Holaigah, I., Rowe, P. C., Kan, J., & Calkins, H. (1995). The relationship between neurally mediated hypotension and the Chronic Fatigue Syndrome. *Journal of the American Medical Association, 274,* 961–967.

Bower, B. (1991). Questions of mind over immunity. *Science News, 139,* 216–217.

Bowling, A. (1991). *Measuring health. A review of quality of life measurement scales.* Philadelphia: Open University.

Brickman, A. L., & Fins, A. I. (1993). Psychological and cognitive aspects of Chronic Fatigue Syndrome. In P. J. Goodnick & N. G. Klimas (Eds.), *Chronic fatigue and related immune deficiency syndromes* (pp. 67–93). Washington, DC: American Psychiatric Press.

Bridges, K. W., & Goldberg, D. P. (1986). The validation of the GHQ and the use of the MMSE in neurological inpatients. *British Journal of Psychiatry, 148,* 548–553.

Briggs, N. C., & Levine, P. H. (1994). A comparative review of systemic and neurological symptomatology in 12 outbreaks collectively described as chronic fatigue syndrome, epidemic neuromyasthenia and myalgic encephalomyelitis. *Clinical Infectious Diseases, 18*(Suppl. 1), S32–S42.

Brook, R. H., Ware, J. E., Davies-Avery, A., Stewart, A. L., Donald, C. A., Rogers, W. H., Williams, K. N., & Johnston, S. A. (1979). Overview of adult health status measures fielded in Rand's health insurance study. *Medical Care, 17*(Suppl. 7), 1–131.

Brouwer, B., & Packer, T. (1994). Corticospinal excitability in patients diagnosed with Chronic Fatigue Syndrome. *Muscle and Nerve, 17,* 1210–1212.

Brown, W. A. (1993). Endocrine correlates of sadness and elation. Psychosomatic *Medicine, 55,* 458–467.

Buchwald, D. (1996). Fibromyalgia and chronic fatigue syndrome: Similarities and differences. *Rheumatic Diseases Clinics of North America, 22,* 219–243.

Buchwald, D., & Garrity, D. (1994). Comparison of patients with chronic fatigue syndrome, fibromyalgia, and multiple chemical sensitivities. *Archives of Internal Medicine, 154,* 2049–2053.

Buchwald, D., Pascualy, R., Bombardier, C., & Kith, P. (1994). Sleep disorders in patients with chronic fatigue syndrome. *Clinical Infectious Diseases, 18*(Suppl. 1), S68–S72.

Buchwald, D., Pearlman, T., Kith, P., Katon, W., & Schmaling, K. (1997). Screening for psychiatric disorders in chronic fatigue and chronic fatigue syndrome. *Journal of Psychosomatic Research, 42,* 87–94.

Buchwald, D., Pearlman, T., Umali, J., Schmaling, K., & Katon, W. (1996). Functional status in patients with chronic fatigue syndrome, other fatiguing illnesses, and healthy individuals. *American Journal of Medicine, 101,* 364–370.

Buchwald, D., Umali, P., Umali, J., Kith, P., Pearlman, T., & Komaroff, A. L. (1995). Chronic fatigue and chronic fatigue syndrome prevalence in a Pacific-Northwest healthcare system. *Annals of Internal Medicine, 123,* 81–88.

Buchwald, H. M., & Rudick-Davis, D. (1993). The symptoms of major depression. *Journal of Abnormal Psychology, 102,* 197–200.

Butler, C., & Rollnick, S. (1996). Missing the meaning and provoking resistance: A case of myalgic encephalomyelitis. *Family Practice, 13,* 106–109.

Butler, S., Chalder, T., Ron, M., & Wessely, S. (1991). Cognitive behavior therapy in chronic fatigue syndrome. *Journal of Neurology, Neurosurgery and Psychiatry, 54,* 153–158.

Calabrese, L. H., Davis, M. E., & Wilke, W. S. (1992, October). *Chronic Fatigue Syndrome (CFS) and Sjogrens Syndrome (SS): An important etiologic relationship.* Paper presented at the meeting of the International CFS/ME Research Conference, Albany, NY.

Camacho, J. A., & Jason, L. A. (1997). *Psychological factors show little relationship to Chronic Fatigue Syndrome recovery.* Manuscript submitted for publication.

Canadian Research Group. (1987). A randomized controlled trial of amantadine in fatigue associated with multiple sclerosis. *Canadian Journal of Neurological Science, 14,* 273–278.

Carpman, V. (1995). The CFIDS treatment: The Cheney clinic's strategic approach. *The CFIDS Chronicle, 8,* 38–45.

Carver, C. S., Scheier, M. F., & Weintraub, J. K. (1989). Assessing coping strategies: A theoretically based approach. *Journal of Personality and Social Psychology, 56,* 267–283.

Centers for Disease Control and Prevention. (1994). *The facts about chronic fatigue syndrome.* Atlanta, GA: U.S. Department of Health and Human Services.

CFIDS News. (1997). Ampligen update. *CFIDS Chronicle, 10,* 25.

Chalder, T., Berelowitz, G., Pawlikowska, J., Watts, L., & Wessely, D. (1993). Development of a fatigue scale. *Journal of Psychosomatic Research, 37,* 147–153.

Chalder, T., Deale, A., & Wessely, S. (1995). Cognitive behavioral therapy for chronic fatigue syndrome [Letter to the editor.] *Clinical Infectious Diseases, 20,* 717.

Chambers, M. J., & Docktor, B. J. (1993). Fatigue scale lacks adequate validation [Letter to the editor]. *Psychiatry Research, 46,* 207–208.

Clark, D. M. (1986). A cognitive approach to panic. *Behavior Research and Therapy, 24,* 461–470.

Clark, K. K., Bormann, C. A., Cropanzano, R. S., & James, K. (1995). Validation evidence for three coping measures. *Journal of Personality Assessment, 65,* 434–455.

Cleare, A. J., Bearn, J., Allain, T., McGregor, A., Wessely, S., Murray, R. M., & O'Keane, V. (1995). Contrasting neuroendocrine responses in depression and chronic fatigue syndrome. *Journal of Affective Disorders, 35,* 283–289.

Clements, A., Sharpe, M., Simkin, S., Borrill, J., & Hawton, K. (1997). Chronic fatigue syndrome—A qualitative investigation of patients' beliefs about the illness. *Journal of Psychosomatic Research, 42,* 615–624.

Cohen, S., & Herbert, T. B. (1996). Health psychology: Psychological factors and physical disease from the perspectives of human psychoneuroimmunology. *Annual Review of Psychology, 47,* 113–142.

Cohen, S., & Williamson, G. M. (1991). Stress and disease in humans. *Psychological Bulletin, 109,* 5–24.

Collinge, W. (1993). *Recovering from Chronic Fatigue Syndrome.* New York: The Body Press/Perigee.

Cope, H., David, A., Pelosi, A., & Mann, A. (1994). Predictors of chronic "postviral" fatigue. *The Lancet, 344,* 864–868.

Cope, H., Mann, A., Pelosi, A., & David, A. (1996). Psychosocial risk factors for chronic fatigue and chronic fatigue syndrome following presumed viral illness: A case-control study. *Psychological Medicine, 26,* 1197–1209.

Cope, H., Pernet, A., Kendall, B., & David, A. (1995). Cognitive functioning and magnetic resonance imaging in chronic fatigue. *British Journal of Psychiatry, 167,* 86–94.

Cordero, D. L., Sisto, S. A., Tapp, W. N., LaManca, J. J., Pareja, J. G., & Natelson, B. H. (1996). Decreased vagal power during treadmill walking in patients with chronic fatigue syndrome. *Clinical Automatic Research, 6,* 329–333.

Cox, I. M., Campbell, M. J., & Dowson, D. (1991). Red blood cell magnesium and chronic fatigue syndrome. *Lancet, 337,* 757–760.

Cripe, L. I., Maxwell, J. K., & Hill, E. (1995). Multivariate discriminant function analysis of neurologic, pain and psychiatric patients with the MMPI. *Journal of Clinical Psychology, 51,* 258–268.

Crisson, J. E., & Keefe, F. J. (1988). The relationship of locus of control to pain coping strategies and psychological distress in chronic pain patients. *Pain, 35,* 147–154.

Croog, S. H., Levine, S., Testa, M. A., Brown, B., Bulpitt, C. J., Jenkins, C. D., Klerman, G. L., & Williams, G. H. (1986). The effects of antihypertensive therapy on quality of life. *New England Journal of Medicine, 314,* 1657–1664.

Cullen, M. R. (1987). The worker with multiple chemical sensitivities: An overview. In M. R. Cullen (Ed.), *Occupational medicine: State of the art reviews* (pp.655–661). Philadelphia: Hanley and Belfus.

Curran, S. L., Andrykowski, M. A., & Studts, J. L. (1983). Short form of the Profile of Mood States (POMS-SF): Psychometric information. *Psychological Assessment, 1,* 80–83.

David, A. S., Wessely, S., & Pelosi, A. J. (1991). Chronic fatigue syndrome: Signs of a new approach. *British Journal of Hospital Medicine, 45,* 158–163.

Davies, K. N., Burn, W. K., McKenzie, F. R., & Brothwell, J. A. (1993). Evaluation of the Hospital Anxiety and Depression Scale as a screening instrument in geriatric medical inpatients. *International Journal of Geriatric Psychiatry, 8,* 165–169.

Davis, T. H., Jason, L. A., & Banghart, M. A. (in press). The effect of housing on individuals with multiple chemical sensitivities. *Journal of Primary Prevention.*

Deale, A., Chalder, T., Marks, I., & Wessely, S. (1997). Cognitive behavior therapy for chronic fatigue syndrome: A randomized controlled trial. *American Journal of Psychiatry, 154,* 408–414.

Dechene, L., Friedberg, F., McKenzie, M., & Fontanetta, R. (1994, October). *A new fatigue typology for Chronic Fatigue Syndrome.* Paper presented at the American Association of Chronic Fatigue Syndrome Research Conference, Ft. Lauderdale, FL.

de Figueiredo, J. M. (1993). Depression and demoralization: Phenomenologic differences and research perspectives. *Comprehensive Psychiatry, 34,* 308–311.

DeLuca, J., Johnson, S. K., Beldowicz, D., & Natelson, B. H. (1995). Neuropsychological performance in chronic fatigue syndrome, multiple sclerosis, and depression. *Journal of Neurology, Neurosurgery, and Psychiatry, 58,* 38–43.

DeLuca, J., Johnson, S. K., & Natelson, B. H. (1995, August). *Are neuropsychological disturbances in chronic fatigue syndrome due to depression?* Paper presented at the 103rd annual convention of the American Psychological Association, New York, NY.

Demitrack, M. A. (1993). Neuroendocrine research strategies in Chronic Fatigue Syndrome. In P. J. Goodnick & N. G. Klimas (Eds.), *Chronic fatigue and related immune deficiency syndromes* (pp. 45–66). Washington, DC: American Psychiatric Press.

Demitrack, M. A., Dale, J. K., Straus, E. E., Lane, L., & Listwak, S. J. (1991). Evidence for impaired activation of the hypothalamic-pituitary-adrenal axis in patients with chronic fatigue syndrome. *Journal of Clinical Endocrinology and Metabolism, 73,* 1224–1234.

Denz-Penhey, H., & Murdoch, J. C. (1993). Service delivery for people with Chronic Fatigue Syndrome: A pilot action research study. *Family Practice, 10,* 14–18.

Derogatis, L. R. (1975). *Brief Symptom Inventory.* Baltimore: Clinical Psychometric Research.

Derogatis, L. R. (1983). *SCL-90-R administration, scoring and procedure manual–II.* Towson, MD: Psychometric Research.

Deyo, R. A., & Inui, T. S. (1983). Measuring functional outcomes in chronic disease: A comparison of traditional scales and a self-administered health status questionnaire in patients with rheumatoid arthritis. *Medical Care, 21,* 180–192.

Deyo, R. A., Inui, T. S., Leininger, J. D., & Overman, S. (1982). Physical and psychological functions in rheumatoid arthritis: Clinical use of a self-administered health status instrument. *Archives of Internal Medicine, 142,* 879–882.

Dobbins, J. G., Natelson, B. H., Brassloff, M. D., Vrastal, S., & Sisto, S. A. (1995). Physical, behavioral and psychological risk factors of chronic fatigue syndrome: A central role for stress? *Journal of Chronic Fatigue Syndrome, 1,* 43–58.

Donati, F., Fagioli, L., Komaroff, A. L., & Duffy, F. H. (1994, October). *Quantified EEG findings in patients with Chronic Fatigue Syndrome.* Paper presented at the American Association of Chronic Fatigue Syndrome Research Conference, Ft. Lauderdale, FL.

Dreher, H. (1995). *The immune power personality.* New York: Dutton.

Drossman, R. A. (1995). Diagnosing and treating patients with refractory functional gastrointestinal symptoms. *Annals of Internal Medicine, 123,* 688–697.

Drossman, R. A., & Thompson, W. G. (1992). The irritable bowel syndrome review as a graded multicomponent treatment approach. *Annals of Internal Medicine, 116,* 1009–1116.

Dunstan, R. H., Donohoe, M., Taylor, W., Roberts, T. K., Murdoch, R. N., Watkins, J. A., & McGregor, N. R. (1995). A preliminary investigation of chlorinated hydrocarbons and chronic fatigue syndrome. *Medical Journal of Australia, 163,* 294–297.

Dutton, D. B. (1986). Social class, health and illness. In L. Aiken & D. Mechanic (Eds.), *Applications of social science to clinical medicine, and health policy* (pp. 31–62). New Brunswick, NJ: Rutgers University Press.

Ehrenreich, B., & English, D. (1989). *For her own good: 150 years of experts' advice to women.* New York: Anchor Books.

Ellis, A. (1962). *Reason and emotion in psychotherapy.* New York: Lyle Stuart.

Ellis, A. (1997). Using rational emotive behavior therapy techniques to cope with disability. *Professional Psychology Research and Practice, 28,* 17–22.

Ellis, A., & Abrams, M. (1994). *How to cope with a fatal illness.* New York: Barricade Books.

Euba, R., Chalder, T., Deale, A., & Wessely, S. (1996). A comparison of the characteristics of Chronic Fatigue Syndrome in primary and tertiary care. *British Journal of Psychiatry, 168,* 121–126.

Farmer, A., Chubb, H., Jones, I., Hillier, J., Smith, A., & Borysiewicz, L. (1996). Screening for psychiatric morbidity in subjects presenting with chronic fatigue syndrome. *British Journal of Psychiatry, 168,* 354–358.

Fawzy, I., Cousins, N., Fawzy, N. W., & Kemeny, M. E. (1990). A structured psychiatric intervention for cancer patients: I. Changes over time in methods of coping and affective disturbance. *Archives of General Psychiatry, 47,* 720–725.

Fechner-Bates, S., Coyne, J. C., & Schwenk, J. L. (1994). The relationship of self-reported distress to depressive disorders and other psychopathology. *Journal of Consulting and Clinical Psychology, 62,* 550–559.

Fennell, P. (1995a). CFS sociocultural influences and trauma: Clinical considerations. *Journal of Chronic Fatigue Syndrome, 1,* 159–173.

Fennell, P. A. (1995b). A four stage progressive model of CFS. *Journal of Chronic Fatigue Syndrome, 1,* 69–79.

Ferrari, J. R., & Jason, L. A. (1997). Caring for people with chronic fatigue syndrome: Perceived stress versus satisfaction. *Rehabilitation Counseling Bulletin, 40,* 240–250.

Field, T. M., Sunshe, W., Hernandez-Reif, M., Quintino, O., Schanberg, S., Kuhn, C., & Burman, I. (1997). Massage therapy effects on depression and somatic symptoms in chronic fatigue syndrome. *Journal of Chronic Fatigue Syndrome, 3,* 43–52.

Fiedler, N., Kipen, H. M., DeLuca, J., Kelly, M., & Natelson, B. (1996). A controlled comparison of multiple chemical sensitivities and chronic fatigue syndrome. *Psychosomatic Medicine, 58,* 38–49.

Finlay-Jones, R. A., & Murphy, E. (1979). Severity of psychiatric disorder and the 30 Item General Health Questionnaire, *British Journal of Psychiatry, 134,* 609–616.

Fischler, B., Cluydts, R., Degucht, V., Kaufman, L., & Demeirleir, K. (1997). Generalized anxiety disorder in chronic fatigue syndrome. *Acta Psychiatrica Scandinavia, 95,* 405–413.

Fischler, B., Dendale, P., Michiels, V., Cluydts, R., Kaufman, L., & Demeirleir, K. (1997). Physical fatigability and exercise capacity in chronic fatigue syndrome— Association with disability, somatization and psychopathology. *Journal of Psychosomatic Research, 42,* 369–378.

Fisk, J. D., Ritvo, P. G., Ross, L., Haase, D. A., & Marrie, T. J. (1994). Measuring the functional impact of fatigue: Initial validation of the Fatigue Impact Scale. *Clinical Infectious Diseases, 18*(Suppl. 1), 579–583.

Folkman, S., & Lazarus, R. (1980). An analysis of coping in a middle aged community sample. *Journal of Health and Social Behaviour, 21,* 219–239.

Fordyce, W. E. (1976). *Behavioral methods for chronic pain and illness.* St. Louis: CV Mosby.

Fowler, F. J., Wennberg, J. E., & Timothy, R. P. (1988). Symptom status and quality of life following prostatectomy. *JAMA, 259,* 3018.

Francis, C. (1990). ME: Time for a break with the past. *Psychiatric Bulletin of the Royal College of Psychiatrists,* (Suppl. 2), 24–25.

Frank, R., Chaney, J., Clay, D. L., Shutty, M. S., Beck, N. C., Kay, D. R., Elliott, T. R., & Grambling, S. (1992). Dysphoria: A major symptom factor in persons with disability or chronic illness. *Psychiatry Research, 43,* 231–241.

Friedberg, F. (1995a, August). *Assessment and treatment of chronic fatigue.* Paper presented at the 103rd annual convention of the American Psychological Association, New York, NY.

Friedberg, F. (1995b). Clinical assessment of coping in chronic fatigue syndrome patients. *Journal of Chronic Fatigue Syndrome, 1,* 53–58.

Friedberg, F. (1995c). *Coping with chronic fatigue syndrome. Nine things you can do.* Oakland, CA: New Harbinger.

Friedberg, F. (1995d). The stress/fatigue link in chronic fatigue syndrome. *Journal of Chronic Fatigue Syndrome, 1,* 147–152.

Friedberg, F. (1996a). Chronic Fatigue Syndrome: A new clinical application. *Professional Psychology: Research and Practice, 27,* 487–494.

Friedberg, F. (1996b, August). *Melancholic depression and chronic fatigue syndrome.* Paper presented at the 104th annual convention of the American Psychological Association, Toronto, Canada.

Friedberg, F., & Jason, L. A. (1998). *A subgrouping scheme for chronic fatigue syndrome.* Unpublished manuscript, State University of New York at Stony Brook.

Friedberg, F., & Krupp, L. B. (1994). A comparison of cognitive behavioral treatment for chronic fatigue syndrome and primary depression. *Clinical Infectious Diseases, 18* (Suppl. 1), S105–S110.

Friedberg, F., & Krupp, L. B. (1995). Cognitive behavioral treatment for chronic fatigue syndrome: Reply [Letter to the editor]. *Clinical Infectious Diseases, 20,* 717–718.

Friedberg, F., McKenzie, M., Dechene, L., & Fontanetta, R. (1994, October). *Symptom patterns in long-term Chronic Fatigue Syndrome.* Paper presented at the American Association of Chronic Fatigue Syndrome Research Conference, Ft. Lauderdale, FL.

Fry, A. M., & Martin, M. (1996). Cognitive idiosyncrasies among children with the Chronic Fatigue Syndrome: Anomalies in self-reported activity levels. *Journal of Psychosomatic Research, 41,* 213–223.

Fukuda, K., Straus, S. E., Hickie, I., Sharpe, M. C., Dobbins, J. G., & Komaroff, A. (1994). The Chronic Fatigue Syndrome: A comprehensive approach to its definition and study. *Annals of Internal Medicine, 121,* 953–959.

Fulcher, K. Y., & White, P. D. (1997). Randomised controlled trial of graded exercise in patients with the chronic fatigue syndrome. *British Medical Journal, 314,* 1647–1652.

Geist, C., & Calzaretta, W. A. (1982). *Placement handbook for counseling disabled persons.* Springfield, IL: Charles C Thomas.

Gellhorn, E. (1968). CNS tuning and its implications for neuropsychiatry. *Journal of Nervous and Mental Diseases, 147,* 148–162.

Gellhorn, E. (1970). The emotions and the ergotropic and trophotropic systems. *Psychologische Forschung, 34,* 48–94.

Gellhorn, E., & Keily, W. F. (1972). Mystical states of consciousness: Neurophysiological and clinical aspects. *Journal of Nervous and Mental Diseases, 154,* 399–405.

Gilman, C. P. (1993). *The yellow wallpaper.* New Brunswick, NJ: Rutgers University Press.

Girdano, D. A., Everly, G. S., Jr., & Dusek, D. E. (1990). *Controlling stress and tension. A holistic approach.* Englewood Cliffs, NJ: Prentice Hall.

Glaser, R., Kiecolt-Glaser, J. K., Speicher, C. E., & Holliday, J. E. (1985). Stress, loneliness, and changes in herpes virus latency. *Journal of Behavioral Medicine, 8,* 249–260.

Gold, D., Bowden, R., Sixbey, J., Riggs, R., Katon, W. J., Ashley, R., Obrigewitch, R., & Corey, L. (1990). Chronic fatigue: A prospective clinical and virologic study. *Journal of the American Medical Association, 264,* 48–53.

Goldberg, D. (1972). *The detection of psychiatric illness by questionnaire.* London: Oxford University Press.

Goldberg, D. P., & Bridges, K. W. (1988). Somatic presentations of psychiatric illness in primary care settings. *Journal of Psychosomatic Research, 32,* 137–144.

Golden, W. L., Gersch, W. D., & Robbins, D. M. (1991). *Psychological treatment of cancer patients.* New York: Pergamon.

Goldenberg, D. L. (1988). Research in fibroymyalgia: Past, present and future. *Journal of Rheumatology, 15,* 992–996.

Goldenberg, D. L., Simms, R. W., Geiger, A., & Komaroff, A. L. (1990). High frequency of fibroymyalgia in patients with chronic fatigue seen in a primary care practice. *Arthritis and Rheumatism, 31,* 381–387.

Goldstein, J. A. (1990). *Chronic Fatigue Syndrome: The struggle for health.* Beverly Hills, CA: Chronic Fatigue Syndrome Institute.

Goodnick, P. J., & Sandoval, R. (1993). Psychotropic treatment of Chronic Fatigue Syndrome and related disorders. *The Journal of Clinical Psychiatry, 54,* 13–20.

Goodwin, S. S. (1997). The marital relationship and health in women with chronic fatigue and immune dysfunction syndrome: Views of wives and husbands. *Nursing Research, 46,* 138–146.

Gram, L. F. (1994). Fluoxetine. *New England Journal of Medicine, 331,* 1354–1361.

Greenberg, M. A., Siegel, K. M., Hatcher, B. A., Dowling, B. A., & Bateman-Cass, B. S. W. (1996, March). *Perceived stigmatization and depression women with fibromyalgia.* Paper presented at the 4th International Congress of Behavioral Medicine, Washington, DC.

Greenfield, S., Fitzcharles, M. A., & Esdaile, J. M. (1992). Reactive fibromyalgia syndrome. *Arthritis and Rheumatism, 35,* 678–681.

Grufferman, S. (1991). Issues and problems in the conduct of epidemiologic research on chronic fatigue syndrome. *Reviews of Infectious Diseases, 13,* S60–S67.

Gunn, W. J., Connell, D. B., & Randall, B. (1993). Epidemiology of chronic fatigue syndrome: The Centers-for-Disease-Control study. In B. R. Bock & J. Whelan (Eds.), *Chronic Fatigue Syndrome* (pp. 83–101). New York: Wiley.

Gurwitt, A., Barrett, S., Brown, S., Butaney, E. C. A., Gorman, B., Kilgore, J. L., O'Grady, E., Potaznick, W., Saltzstein, B., Sanford, A., Webster, W., & Zimmer, V. (1992). *Chronic fatigue syndrome: A primer for physicians and allied health professionals.* Waltham, MA: CFIDS Association.

Guthrie, P. C., & Mobley, B. D. (1994). A comparison of the differential diagnostic efficiency of three personality disorder inventories. *Journal of Clinical Psychology, 50,* 656–665.

Halfaway, S. R., & McKinley, J. C. (1940). A multiphasic personality schedule: Construction of the schedule. *Journal of Psychology, 10,* 249–254.

Halfaway, S. R., & McKinley, J. C. (1989). *MMPI-II.* Minneapolis, MN: University of Minnesota Press.

Hamilton, M. (1967). Development of a rating scale for primary depressive illness. *British Journal of Social and Clinical Psychology, 6,* 278–296.

Harkapaa, K., Jarvikoski, A., Mellin, G., Hurri, H., & Luoma, J. (1991). Health locus of control beliefs and psychological distress as predictors for treatment outcome in low-back pain patients: Results of a 3-month follow-up of a controlled intervention study. *Pain, 46,* 35–41.

Hay, L. L. (1984). *You can heal your life.* Carson, CA: Hay House.

Hedrick, T. E. (1997). Summary of risk factors for chronic fatigue syndrome is misleading [Letter to the editor]. *Quarterly Journal of Medicine 90,* 723–725.

Heiman, T. (1994, October). *Chronic Fatigue Syndrome and vocational rehabilitation: Unserved and unmet needs.* Paper presented at the American Association of Chronic Fatigue Syndrome Research Conference, Ft. Lauderdale, FL.

Hickie, I., Lloyd, A., Wakefield, D., & Parker, G. (1990). The psychiatric status of patients with Chronic Fatigue Syndrome. *British Journal of Psychiatry, 156*, 534–540.

Hickie, I., Lloyd, A., Wilson, A., Hadzi-Pavlovic, D., Parker, G., Bird, K., & Wakefield, D. (1995). Can the Chronic Fatigue Syndrome be defined by distinct clinical features? *Psychological Medicine, 25*, 925–935.

Ho-Yen, D.O., & McNamara, I. (1991). General practitioners' experience of the chronic fatigue syndrome. *British Journal of General Practice, 41*, 324–326.

Holmes, G. P. (1991). Defining the Chronic Fatigue Syndrome. *Reviews of Infectious Diseases, 13*, S53–S55.

Holmes, G. P., Kaplan, J. E., Gantz, N. M., Komaroff, A. L., Schonberger, L. B., Straus, S. S., Jones, J. F., Dubois, R. E., Cunningham-Rundles, C., Pahwa, S., Tosato, G., Zegans, L. S., Purtilo, D. T., Brown, W., Schooley, R. T., & Brus, I. (1988). Chronic Fatigue Syndrome: A working case definition. *Annals of Internal Medicine, 108*, 387–389.

Holmes, G. P., Kaplan, J. E., Schonberger, L. B., Straus, S. E., Zegans, L. S., Gantz, N. M., Brus, I., Komaroff, H., Jones, J. F., DuBois, R. E., Cunningham-Rundles, C., Tosato, G., Brown, N. A., Pahwa, S., & Schooley, R. T. (1988). Definition of Chronic Fatigue Syndrome [Letter to the editor]. *Annals of Internal Medicine, 109*, 512.

Huber, S., Freidenberg, D., Paulson, G., Shuttleworth, E., & Christy, J. (1990). The pattern of depressive symptoms varies with progression of Parkinson's disease. *Journal of Neurology, Neurosurgery and Psychiatry, 53*, 275–278.

Iger, L. (1992, Summer). Iger neurocognitive assessment. *The CFIDS Chronicle*, 73–74.

Imboden, J. B., Canter, A., & Cluff, L. E. (1961). Convalescence from influenza: A study of the psychological and clinical determinants. *Archives of Internal Medicine, 108*, 115–121.

James, L. C., & Folen, R. A. (1996). EEG biofeedback as a treatment for chronic fatigue syndrome: A controlled case report. *Behavioral Medicine, 22*, 77–81.

Jamner, L. D., & Schwartz, G. E. (1986). Self-deception predicts self-report and endurance of pain. *Psychosomatic Medicine, 48*, 211–223.

Jamner, L. D., Schwartz, G. E., & Leigh, H. (1988). The relationship between repressive and defensive coping styles and monocyte, eosinophile, and serum glucose levels: Support for the opioid peptide hypothesis of repression. *Psychosomatic Medicine, 50*, 567–575.

Jason, L. A., Ferrari, J. R., Taylor, R. R., Slavich, S. P., & Stenzel, C. L. (1996). A national assessment of the service, support, and housing preferences by persons with Chronic Fatigue Syndrome: Toward a comprehensive rehabilitation program. *Evaluation and the Health Professions, 19*, 194–207.

Jason, L. A., Fitzgibbon, G., Taylor, S. L., Johnson, S., & Salina, D. (1993). Strategies in identifying people with Chronic Fatigue Syndrome. *Journal of Community Psychology, 21*, 339–344.

Jason, L. A., Fitzgibbon, G., Taylor, R., Taylor, S., Wagner, L., Johnson, S., Richmond, G. W., Papernik, M., Plioplys, A. V., Plioplys, S., Lipkin, D., & Ferrari, J. (1993, Summer). The prevalence of Chronic Fatigue Syndrome: A review of efforts—past and present. *The CFIDS Chronicle*, pp. 24–29.

Jason, L. A., Holden, J., Taylor, S. L., & Melrose, H. (1995). Monitoring energy levels in Chronic Fatigue Syndrome. *The Psychological Record, 45*, 643–654.

Jason, L. A., King, C. P., Frankenberry, E. L., Jordan, K. M., & Tryon, W. W. (1998). *Chronic Fatigue Syndrome: Assessing symptoms and activity level.* Manuscript submitted for publication.

Jason, L. A., King, C. P., Tryon, W. W., Frankenberry, E. L., & Jordan, K. M. (1997). *Monitoring and assessing symptoms of Chronic Fatigue Syndrome: Use of time series regression.* Manuscript submitted for publication.

Jason, L. A., Kolak, A. M., Cantillon, D., Purnell, T., Camacho, J. M., Klein, S., & Lerman, A. (1998). *Disability as the lens for new perspectives on community interventions.* Manuscript submitted for publication.

Jason, L. A., Richman, J. A., Friedberg, F., Wagner, L., Taylor, R., & Jordan, K. M. (1997). Politics, science, and the emergence of a new disease: The case of Chronic Fatigue Syndrome. *American Psychologist, 52,* 973–983.

Jason, L. A., Ropacki, M. T., Santoro, N. B., Richman, J. A., Heatherly, W., Taylor, R., Ferrari, J. R., Haney-Davis, T. M., Rademaker, A., Dupuis, J., Golding, J., Plioplys, A. V., & Plioplys, S. (1997). A screening instrument for Chronic Fatigue Syndrome: Reliability and validity. *Journal of Chronic Fatigue Syndrome, 3,* 39–59.

Jason, L. A., & Taylor, S. L. (1994). Monitoring Chronic Fatigue Syndrome. *Journal of Nervous and Mental Disease, 182,* 243–244.

Jason, L. A., Taylor, S. L., Johnson, S., Goldston, S. E., Salina, D., Bishop, P., & Wagner, L. (1993a). Estimating Chronic Fatigue Syndrome-related symptoms among nurses: A preliminary report [Abstract]. *Clinical Infectious Diseases, 18,* S54.

Jason, L. A., Taylor, S. L., Johnson, S., Goldston, S. E., Salina, D., Bishop, P., & Wagner, L. (1993b). Prevalence of Chronic Fatigue Syndrome-related symptoms among nurses. *Evaluation and the Health Professions, 16,* 385–399.

Jason, L. A., Taylor, R., Wagner, L., Holden, J., Ferrari, J. R., Plioplys, A. V., Plioplys, S., Lipkin, D., & Papernik, M. (1995). Estimating rates of Chronic Fatigue Syndrome from a community based sample: A pilot study. *American Journal of Community Psychology, 23,* 557–568.

Jason, L. A., Tryon, W. W., Frankenberry, E. L., & King, C. P. (1997). Chronic Fatigue Syndrome: Relationship of self-ratings and actigraphy. *Psychological Reports, 81,* 1223–1226.

Jason, L. A., Wagner, L., Rosenthal, S., Goodlatte, J., Lipkin, D., Papernik, M., Plioplys, S., & Plioplys, A. V. (in press). Estimating the prevalence of chronic fatigue syndrome among nurses. *American Journal of Medicine.*

Jason, L. A., Wagner, L., Taylor, R., Ropacki, M. T., Shlaes, J., Ferrari, J., Slavich, S. P., & Stenzel, C. (1995). Chronic Fatigue Syndrome: A new challenge for health care professionals. *Journal of Community Psychology, 23,* 143–164.

Johnson, H. (1995). *Osler's web. Inside the labyrinth of Chronic Fatigue Syndrome epidemic.* New York: Crown.

Johnson, S. K., DeLuca, J., & Natelson, B. H. (1996a). Assessing somatization disorder in the Chronic Fatigue Syndrome. *Psychosomatic Medicine, 58,* 50–57.

Johnson, S. K., DeLuca, J., & Natelson, B. H. (1996b). Depression in fatiguing illness: Comparing patients with chronic fatigue syndrome, multiple sclerosis and depression. *Journal of Affective Disorders, 39,* 21–30.

Johnson, S. K., DeLuca, J., & Natelson, B. H. (1996c). Personality dimensions in the Chronic Fatigue Syndrome: A comparison with multiple sclerosis and depression. *Journal of Psychiatric Research, 30,* 9–20.

Joyce, J., Hotopf, M., & Wessely, S. (1997). The prognosis of chronic fatigue and chronic fatigue syndrome: A systematic review. *Quarterly Journal of Medicine, 90,* 223–233.

Kaplan, H. B. (1991). Social psychology of the immune system: A conceptual framework and review of the literature. *Social Science Medicine, 33,* 909–923.

Karnofsky, D. A., Abelmann, W. H., Craver, L. F., & Burchenal, J. H. (1948). The use of nitrogen mustards in the palliative treatment of carcinoma. *Cancer, 1,* 634–656.

Karoly, P., & Jensen, M. P. (1987). *Multimethod assessment of chronic pain.* Oxford, England: Pergamon.

Kasl, S. V., Evans, A. S., & Niederman, J. C. (1979). Psychosocial risk factors in the development of infectious mononucleosis. *Psychosomatic Medicine, 41,* 445–466.

Kaslow, J. E., Rucker, L., & Onishi, R. (1989). Liver extract folic acid-cyanocobalamin vs. placebo for chronic fatigue syndrome. *Archives of Internal Medicine, 149,* 2501–2503.

Katon, W. J., Buchwald, D. S., Simon, G. E., Russo, J. E., & Mease, P. J. (1991). Psychiatric illness in patients with chronic fatigue and rheumatoid arthritis. *Journal of General Internal Medicine, 6,* 277–285.

Katon, W., & Russo, J. (1992). Chronic Fatigue Syndrome criteria. A critique of the requirement for multiple physical complaints. *Archives of Internal Medicine, 152,* 1604–1609.

Katon, W., & Walker, E. A. (1993). The relationship of chronic fatigue to psychiatric illness in community, primary care and tertiary care samples. In B. R. Bock & J. Whelan (Eds.), *Chronic fatigue syndrome* (pp. 193–211). New York: Wiley.

Keefe, F. J., Dunsmore, J., & Burnet, R. (1992). Behavioral and cognitive behavioral approaches to chronic pain: Recent advances and future directions. *Journal of Consulting and Clinical Psychology, 60,* 528–536.

Kelly, J. G. (1985). The concept of primary prevention: Creating new paradigms. *Journal of Primary Prevention, 5,* 269–272.

Kelly, J. G. (1987, April). *Beyond prevention techniques: Generating social settings for a public's health.* Paper presented at the Tenth Erich Lindemann Memorial Lecture, Harvard Medical School, Boston, MA.

Kerns, R. D., Turk, D. C., & Rudy, T. E. (1985). The West Haven–Yale Multidimensional Pain Inventory (WHYMPI). *Pain, 23,* 345–356.

Kiecolt-Glaser, J. K., Fisher, L., Ogrocks, P., Stout, J. C., & Speicher, C. E. (1987). Marital quality, marital disruption, and immune function. *Psychosomatic Medicine, 49,* 13–34.

Kiecolt-Glaser, J. K., Garner, W., Speicher, C. E., Penn, G., & Glaser, R. (1984). Psychosocial modifiers of immunocompetence in medical students. *Psychosomatic Medicine, 46,* 7–14.

Kiecolt-Glaser, J. K., & Glaser, R. (1989). Psychoneuroimmunology: Past, present, and future. *Health Psychology, 8,* 677–682.

Kiecolt-Glaser, J. K., & Glaser, R. (1992). Psychoneuroimmunology: Can psychological interventions modulate immunity? *Journal of Consulting and Clinical Psychology, 60,* 569–575.

King, C. P., Jason, L. A., Frankenberry, E. L., Jordan, K. M., & Tryon, W. (1997). Managing chronic fatigue syndrome through behavioral monitoring of energy levels and fatigue: A case study demonstrating the envelope theory. *CFIDS Chronicle, 10,* 10–14.

Klein, A. (1989). *The healing power of humor.* Los Angeles, CA: Jeremy P. Tarcher.

Klonoff, D. C. (1992). Chronic fatigue syndrome. *Clinical Infectious Diseases, 15,* 812–823.

Kobasa, S. C., Maddi, S. R., Puccetti, M. C., & Zola, M. A. (1985). Effectiveness of hardiness, exercise, and social support as resources against illness. *Journal of Psychosomatic Research, 29,* 525–533.

Kodama, M., Kodama, T., & Murakami, M. (1996). The value of the dehydro-epiandrosterone-annexed vitamin C infusion treatment in the clinical control of chronic fatigue syndrome (CFS). II. Characterization of CFS patients with special reference to their response to a new vitamin C infusion treatment. *In Vivo, 10,* 585–596.

Komaroff, A. L., & Buchwald, D. (1991). Symptoms and signs of Chronic Fatigue Syndrome. *Review of Infectious Diseases, 13,* S8–S11.

Komaroff, A. L., Fagioli, L. R., Geiger, A. M., Doolittle, T. H., Lee, J., Kornish, R. J., Gleit, M. A., & Guerriero, R. T. (1996). An examination of the working case definition of chronic fatigue syndrome. *American Journal of Medicine, 100,* 56–64.

Komaroff, A. L., & Geiger, A. (1989). Does the CDC working case definition of chronic fatigue syndrome identify a distinct group? [Abstract]. *Clinical Research, 37,* 778A.

Kritchevsky, D. (1995). Diet in heart disease and cancer. *Advances in Experimental Medicine & Biology, 369,* 201–209.

Kroenke, K., Wood, D., Mangelsdorff, D., Meier, N., & Powell, J. (1988). Chronic fatigue in primary care: Prevalence, patient characteristics and outcome. *Journal of the American Medical Association, 260,* 929–934.

Kruesi, M. J., Dale, J., & Straus, S. E. (1989). Psychiatric diagnosis in patients who have chronic fatigue syndrome. *Journal of Clinical Psychiatry, 50,* 53–56.

Krupp, L. B., La Rocca, N. G., Muir-Nash, J., & Steinberg, A. D. (1989). The Fatigue Severity Scale: Application to patients with multiple sclerosis and systemic lupus erythematosis. *Archives of Neurology, 46,* 1121–1123.

Krupp, L. B., & Mendelson, W. B. (1990). Sleep disorders in chronic fatigue syndrome. In J. Horne (Ed.) *Sleep '90* (pp. 261–263). Bochum, Germany: Pontenagel Press.

Krupp, L. B., Mendelson, W. B., & Friedman, R. (1991). An overview of Chronic Fatigue Syndrome. *Journal of Clinical Psychiatry, 52,* 403–410.

Krupp, L. B., Sliwinski, M., Masur, D. M., Friedberg, F., & Coyle, P. K. (1994). Cognitive functioning and depression in patients with chronic fatigue syndrome

and multiple sclerosis. *Archives of Neurology, 57,* 705–710.

Landay, A. L., Jessop, C., Lennette, E. T., & Levy, J. A. (1991). Chronic fatigue syndrome: Clinical condition associated with immune activation. *Lancet, 338,* 707–712.

Lane, T. J., Manu, P., & Matthews, D. A. (1991). Depression and somatization in the Chronic Fatigue Syndrome. *American Journal of Medicine, 91,* 335–344.

Lanham, R. J., & Lanham, J. H. (1994, October). *Autoimmune diseases (auto) in the families of patients (PTs) with Chronic Fatigue Syndrome (CFS) in Western New York (WNY).* Paper presented at the American Association of Chronic Fatigue Syndrome Research Conference, Ft. Lauderdale, FL.

Lawrie, S. M., & Pelosi, A. J. (1995). Chronic Fatigue Syndrome in the community. Prevalence and associations. *British Journal of Psychiatry, 166,* 793–797.

Lawson, L. (1993). *Staying well in a toxic world.* Chicago: Noble Press.

Lazarus, A. A. (1976). *Multimodal behavior therapy.* New York: Springer.

Lee, K. A., Hicks, G., & Nino-Murcia, G. (1991). Validity and reliability of a scale to assess fatigue. *Psychiatry Research, 36,* 291–298.

Leese, G., Chattington, P., Fraser, W., Vora, J., Edwards, R., & Williams, G. (1996). Short-term night-shift working mimics the pituitary-adrenocortical dysfunction in chronic fatigue syndrome. *Journal of Clinical Endocrinology and Metabolism, 81,* 1867–1870.

LeRoy, J., Haney Davis, T., & Jason, L. A. (1996). Treatment efficacy: A survey of 305 MCS patients. *CFIDS Chronicle, 9,* 52–53.

Lewis, S., Cooper, C. L., & Bennett, D. (1994). Psychosocial factors and chronic fatigue syndrome. *Psychological Medicine, 24,* 661–671.

Lipkin, D. M., Robin, R., Vasques, L., Plioplys, A. K., & Plioplys, S. (1995).

Chronic fatigue syndrome [Letter to the editor]. *Journal of Neurology, Neurosurgery & Psychiatry, 58,* 764–765.

Lloyd, A. R., Hickie, I., Boughton, C. R., Spencer, O., & Wakefield, D. (1990). Prevalence of chronic fatigue syndrome in an Australian population. *Medical Journal of Australia, 153,* 522–528.

Lloyd, A. R., Hickie, I., Brockman, A., Hickie, C., Wilson, A., Dwyer, J., & Wakefield, D. (1993). Immunologic and psychologic therapy for patients with Chronic Fatigue Syndrome: A double-blind, placebo-controlled trial. *American Journal of Medicine, 94,* 197–203.

Lutgendorf, S. K., Antoni, M. H., Ironson, G., Fletcher, M. A., Penedo, F., Baum, A., Schneiderman, N., & Klimas, N. (1995). Physical symptoms of Chronic Fatigue Syndrome are exacerbated by the stress of Hurricane Andrew. *Psychosomatic Medicine, 57,* 310–323.

Lutgendorf, S., Klimas, N. G., Antoni, M., Brickman, A., & Fletcher, M. A. (1995). Relationships of cognitive difficulties to immune measures, depression and illness burden in Chronic Fatigue Syndrome. *Journal of Chronic Fatigue Syndrome, 1,* 23–41.

Lydiard, R. B., Fossey, M. D., Marsh, W., & Ballenger, J. C. (1993). Prevalence of psychiatric disorders in patients with irritable bowel syndrome. *Psychosomatic, 34,* 229–234.

Lynch, S., Seth, R., & Montgomery, S. (1990). The use of antidepressant therapy in the chronic fatigue syndrome. *Psychiatric Bulletin of the Royal College of Psychiatrists* (Suppl. 3), 43.

MacDonald, K. L., Osterholm, M. T., LeDell, K. H., White, K. E., & Schenk, C. H. (1996). A case-control study to assess possible triggers and cofactors in chronic fatigue syndrome. *American Journal of Medicine, 100,* 548–554.

Maier, S. F., Watkins, L. R., & Fleshner, M. (1994). Psychoneuroimmunology: The interface between behavior, brain, and immunity. *American Psychologist, 49,* 1004–1017.

Main, C. J. (1983). The Modified Somatic Perception Questionnaire (MSPQ). *Journal of Psychosomatic Research, 27,* 503–514.

Main, C. J., & Waddell, G. (1987). Psychometric construction and validity of the Pilowsky Illness Behavior Questionnaire in British patients with chronic low back pain. *Pain, 28,* 13–25.

Manu, P., Lane, T. J., & Matthews, D. A. (1988). The frequency of the Chronic Fatigue Syndrome in patients with symptoms of persistent fatigue. *Annals of Internal Medicine, 109,* 554–556.

Manu, P., Lane, T. J., & Matthews, D. A. (1992a). Chronic Fatigue Syndromes in clinical practice. *Psychotherapy Psychosomatics, 58,* 60–68.

Manu, P., Lane, T. J., & Matthews, D. A. (1992b). The pathophysiology of chronic fatigue syndrome: Confirmations, contradictions, and conjectures. *International Journal of Psychiatry in Medicine, 22,* 397–408.

Manu, P., Matthews, D., & Lane, T. (1988). The mental health of patients with a chief complaint of chronic fatigue: A prospective evaluation and follow-up. *Archives of Internal Medicine, 148,* 2213–2217.

Manu, P., Matthews, D., Lane, T., Tennen, H., Hesselbrock, V., Mendola, R., & Affleck, G. (1989). Depression among patients with a chief complaint of chronic fatigue. *Journal of Affective Disorders, 17,* 165–172.

Manuck, S. B., Cohen, S., Rabin, B. S., Muldoon, M. F., & Bachen, E. A. (1991). Individual differences in cellular immune response to stress. *Psychological Science, 2,* 111–115.

Martinson, E. W. (1987). The role of aerobic exercise in the treatment of depression. *Stress Medicine, 3,* 93–110.

Maton, K. I. (1989). Towards an ecological understanding of mutual-help groups:

The social ecology of *fit.* *American Journal of Community Psychology, 17,* 729–753.

Mattlin, J. A., Wethington, E., & Kessler, R. C. (1990). Situational determinants of coping and coping effectiveness. *Journal of Health & Social Behavior, 31,* 103–122.

McBride, J. J., & McCluskey, D. R. (1991). Treatment of chronic fatigue syndrome. *British Medical Bulletin, 47,* 895–907.

McCann, J. T. (1990). A multitrait, multimethod analysis of the MCMI-II Clinical Syndrome Scales. *Journal of Personality Assessment, 55,* 465–476.

McClelland, D. C., Floor, E., Davidson, R. J., & Saron, S. (1980). Stressed power motivation, sympathetic activation, immune function, and illness. *Journal of Human Stress, 6,* 11–19.

McCluskey, D. R. (1993). Pharmacological approaches to the therapy of chronic fatigue syndrome. In B. R. Bock & J. Whelan (Eds.), *Chronic Fatigue Syndrome* (pp. 280–297). New York: Wiley.

McHorney, C. A., Ware, J. E., & Raczek, A. E. (1993). The MOS 36-Item Short-Form Health Survey (SF-36): II. Psychometric and clinical tests of validity in measuring physical and mental health constructs. *Medical Care, 31,* 247–263.

McHorney, C. A., Ware, J. E., Wu, A. W., & Sherbourne, C. D. (1994). The MOS 36-Item Short-Form Health Survey (SF-36): III. Tests of data quality, scaling assumptions, and reliability across diverse patient groups. *Medical Care, 32,* 40–66.

McKenzie, M., Dechene, L., Friedberg, F., & Fontanetta, R. (1995). Cognitive–behavioral coping skills in long-term chronic fatigue syndrome. *Journal of Chronic Fatigue Syndrome, 1,* 59–67.

McLean, J., & Pietroni, P. (1990). Self-care: Who does best? *Social Science and Medicine, 30,* 591–596.

McNair, D., Lorr, R. & Droppleman, L. (1992). *Edits manual for the Profile of Mood States.* San Diego, CA: Educational and Industrial Testing Services.

Mechanic, D. (1983). The experience and expression of distress: The study of illness behavior and medical utilization. In D. Mechanic (Ed.), *Handbook of health care and the health professions* (pp. 591–607). New York: Free Press.

Melzack, R. (1983). The McGill Pain Questionnaire. In R. Melzack (Ed.), *Pain management and assessment* (pp. 41–48), New York: Raybin Press.

Meyer, R., & Haggarty, R. (1962). Streptococcal infections in families. *Pediatrics,* 539–549.

Miller, J. F. (1992). *Coping with chronic illness: Overcoming powerlessness.* Philadelphia: Davis.

Millon, C., Fernando, S., Blaney, N., Morgan, R., & Mantero-Atienza, E. (1989). A psychological assessment of chronic fatigue syndrome/chronic Epstein–Barr virus patients. *Psychology and Health: An International Journal, 3,* 131–141.

Millon, T. (1987). *Millon Clinical Multiaxial Inventory–II, manual* (2nd ed.). Minneapolis, MN: National Computer Systems.

Millon, T., Millon, C., & Davis, R. D. (1994). Millon Clinical Multiaxial Inventory–III. Minneapolis, MN: National Computer Systems.

Montague, T. R., Marie, T. I., Klassen, G. A., Bewick, D. J., & Horacek, B. M. (1989). Cardiac function at rest and with exercise in the chronic fatigue syndrome. *Chest, 95,* 779–784.

Montgomery, G. K. (1983). Uncommon tiredness among college undergraduates. *Journal of Consulting and Clinical Psychology, 51,* 517–525.

Mor, V., Lalibert, L., Morris, J. N., & Wienmann, M. (1984). The Karnofsky Performance Status Scale: An examination of its reliability and validity in a research setting. *Cancer, 53,* 2002–2007.

Morrison, T. L., Edwards, D. W., & Weissman, H. N. (1994). The MMPI and

MMPI-II as predictors of psychiatric diagnosis in an outpatient sample. *Journal of Personality Assessment, 62,* 17–30.

Morriss, R., Sharpe, M., Sharpley, A. L., & Hawton, K. (1993). Abnormalities of sleep in patients with the chronic fatigue syndrome. *British Medical Journal, 306,* 1161–1164.

Morriss, R. K., Wearden, A. J., & Battersby, L. (1997). The relation of sleep difficulties to fatigue, mood and disability in chronic fatigue syndrome. *Journal of Psychosomatic Research, 42,* 597–605.

Muscio, B. (1921). Is a fatigue test possible? *British Journal of Psychology, 12,* 31–46.

Natelson, B. H., Cheu, J., Pareja, J., Ellis, S. P., Policastro, T., & Findley, T. W. (1996). Randomized, double blind, controlled placebo-phase in trial of low dose phenelzine in the chronic fatigue syndrome. *Psychopharmacology, 124,* 226–230.

Natelson, B. H., Johnson, S. K., DeLuca, J., Sisto, S., Ellis, S. P., Hill, N., & Bergen, M. J. (1995). Reducing heterogeneity in chronic fatigue syndrome: A comparison with depression and multiple sclerosis. *Clinical Infectious Diseases, 21,* 1204–1210.

Nielson, W. R., Walker, C., & McCain, G. A. (1992). Cognitive–behavioral treatment of fibromyalgia syndrome. *Journal of Rheumatology, 19,* 98–103.

Nocton, J. T., & Steere, J. C. (1995). Lyme disease. *Advances in Internal Medicine, 40,* 69–117.

Ormel, J., Koeter, M. W., & van den Brink, W. (1989). Measuring change with the General Health Questionnaire (GHQ). The problem of retest effects. *Social Psychiatry and Psychiatric Epidemiology, 24,* 227–232.

Packer, T. L., Sauriol, A., & Brouwer, B. (1994). Fatigue secondary to chronic illness: Postpolio syndrome, chronic fatigue syndrome, and multiple sclerosis. *Archives of Physical Medicine and Rehabilitation, 75,* 1122–1126.

Patarca, R., Fletcher, M. A., & Klimas, N. G. (1993). Immunological correlates of Chronic Fatigue Syndrome. In P. J. Goodnick & N. G. Klimas (Eds.), *Chronic fatigue and related immune deficiency syndromes* (pp. 1–21). Washington, DC: American Psychiatric Press.

Pawlikowska, T., Chalder, T., Wessely, S., Wright, D., Hirsch, S., & Wallace, P. (1994). A population based study of fatigue and psychological distress. *British Medical Journal, 308,* 763–766.

Pennebaker, J. W. (1982). *The psychology of physical symptoms.* New York: Springer-Verlag.

Pennebaker, J. W. (1995). Emotion, disclosure, and health: An overview. In J. W. Pennebaker (Ed.), *Emotion, disclosure, and health* (pp. 3–10). Washington, DC: American Psychological Association.

Pennebaker, J. W., & Beall, S. K. (1986). Confronting a traumatic event: Toward an understanding of inhibition and disease. *Journal of Abnormal Psychology, 95,* 274–281.

Pennebaker, J. W., Kiecolt-Glaser, J. K., & Glaser, R. (1988). Disclosure of traumas and immune function: Health implications for psychotherapy. *Journal of Consulting and Clinical Psychology, 56,* 239–245.

Pepper, C. M., Krupp, L. B., Friedberg, F., Doscher, C., & Coyle, P. K. (1993). A comparison of neuropsychiatric characteristics in chronic fatigue syndrome, multiple sclerosis, and major depression. *Journal of Neuropsychiatry and Clinical Neurosciences, 5,* 200–205.

Petrie, K., Moss-Morris, R., & Weinman, J. (1995). The impact of catastrophic beliefs on functioning in chronic fatigue syndrome. *Journal of Psychosomatic Research, 39,* 31–37.

Philips, H. (1987). Avoidance behavior and its role in sustaining chronic pain. *Behaviour Research and Therapy, 25,* 273–279.

Pilowsky, I. (1993). Dimensions of illness behavior as measured by the Illness

Behavior Questionnaire: A replication study. *Journal of Psychosomatic Research, 37*, 53–62.

Pilowsky, I., Spence, N., Cobb, J., & Katsikitis, M. (1984). The Illness Behavior Questionnaire as an aid to clinical assessment. *General Hospital Psychiatry, 6*, 123–130.

Piper, B., Lindsey, A., Dodd, M., Ferketich, S., & Paul, S. (1989). The development of an instrument to measure the subjective dimension of fatigue. In S. Funk, E. Tornquist, M. Champagne, L. Copp, & R. Wiese (Eds.), *Key aspects of comfort: Management of pain, fatigue, and nausea* (pp. 199–207). New York: Springer.

Plioplys, A. V., & Plioplys, S. (1997). Amantadine and L-carnitine treatment of chronic fatigue syndrome. *Neuropsychobiology, 35*, 16–23.

Plumb, M., & Holland, J. (1977). Comparative studies of psychological function in patients with advanced cancer. I. Self-report depressive symptoms. *Psychosomatic Medicine, 39*, 264–276.

Podell, R. N. (1987). *Doctor, why am I so tired?* New York: Pharos Books.

Powell, R., Dolan, R., & Wessely, S. (1990). Attribution and self-esteem in depression and chronic fatigue syndrome. *Journal of Psychosomatic Research, 34*, 65–76.

Price, R. K., North, C. S., Wessely, S., & Fraser, V. J. (1992). Estimating the prevalence of chronic fatigue syndrome and associated symptoms in the community. *Public Health Reports, 107*, 514–522.

Procideno, M. E., & Heller, K. (1983). Measures of perceived social support from friends and from family: Three validated studies. *American Journal of Community of Psychology, 11*, 1–24.

Radloff, L. S. (1977). The CES-D Scale: A self-report depression scale for research in the general population. *Applied Psychological Measurement, 1*, 385–401.

Ray, C. (1991). Chronic fatigue syndrome: Conceptual and methodological ambiguities. *Psychological Medicine, 21*, 1–9.

Ray, C. (1992). Positive and negative social support in a chronic illness. *Psychological Reports, 71*, 977–978.

Ray, C., Jefferies, S., & Weir, W. R. C. (1995a). Coping with chronic fatigue syndrome: Illness responses and their relationship with fatigue, functional impairment and emotional status. *Psychological Medicine, 25*, 937–945.

Ray, C., Jefferies, S., & Weir, W. R. C. (1995b). Life-events and the course of chronic fatigue syndrome. *British Journal of Medical Psychology, 68*, 323–331.

Ray, C., Jefferies, S., & Weir, W. R. C. (1997). Coping and other predictors of outcome in chronic fatigue syndrome. A 1-year follow-up. *Journal of Psychosomatic Research, 43*, 405–415.

Ray, C., Weir, W., Cullen, S., & Phillips, S. (1992). Illness perception and symptom components in chronic fatigue syndrome. *Journal of Psychosomatic Research, 36*, 243–256.

Ray, C., Weir, W. R. C., Phillips, S., & Cullen, S. (1992). Development of a measure of symptoms in chronic fatigue syndrome: The Profile of Fatigue-Related Symptoms (PFRS). *Psychology and Health, 7*, 27–43.

Ray, C., Weir, W., Stewart, D., Miller, P., & Hyde, G. (1993). Ways of coping with chronic fatigue syndrome: Development of an illness management questionnaire. *Social Science Medicine, 37*, 385–391.

Rebouche, C. J., & Engel, A. G. (1983). Carnitine metabolism and deficiency syndromes. *Mayo Clinic Proceedings, 58*, 533–540.

Regier, D. A., Boyd, J. H., Burke, J. D., Jr., Rae, D. S., Myers, J. K., Kramer, M., Robins, L. N., George, L. K., Karno, M., & Locke, B. Z. (1988). One-month prevalence of mental disorders in the United States: Based on five Epidemiological Catchment Area sites. *Archives of General Psychiatry, 45*, 977–986.

Register, C. (1987). Living with chronic illness: Days of patience and passion. New York: Free Press.

Rehabilitation Act Amendment of 1992, Pub. L. No. 102–569. 1992 Amendment to the Rehabilitation Act of 1973.

Report of a joint working group of the Royal Colleges of Physicians, Psychiatrists and General Practitioners. (1996). *Chronic Fatigue Syndrome*. London, Great Britain: Royal College of Physicians, Royal College of Psychiatrists, and Royal College of General Practitioners.

Rhoten, D. (1982). Fatigue and the postsurgical patient. In D. M. Norris (Ed.), *Concept clarification in nursing* (pp. 277–300). Rockville, MD: Aspen Publishers.

Richman, J. A., Flaherty, J. A., & Rospenda, K. M. (1994). Chronic Fatigue Syndrome: Have flawed assumptions derived from treatment-based studies? *American Journal of Public Health, 84,* 282–284.

Rief, W., & Fichter, M. (1992). The Symptom Check List SCL–90–R and its ability to discriminate between dysthymia, anxiety disorders, and anorexia nervosa. *Psychopathology, 25,* 128–138.

Robbins, J. M., Kirmayer, L. J., & Hemami, S. (1997). Latent variable models of functional somatic distress. *Journal of Nervous & Mental Disease, 185,* 606–615.

Robins, L. N., Helzer, J., Cottler, L., & Goldring, E. (1989). *National Institute of Mental Health Diagnostic Interview Schedule, Version Three Revised. DIS–III–R.* St. Louis, MO: Department of Psychiatry, Washington University School of Medicine.

Robins, L. N., & Regier, D. A. (1991). *Psychiatric disorders in America: The ECA study.* New York: Free Press.

Salit, I. E., (1997). Precipitating factors for the chronic fatigue syndrome. *Journal of Psychiatric Research, 31,* 59–65.

Samii, A., Wasserman, E. M., Ikoma, K., Mercuri, B., George, M. S., O'Fallon, A.,

Dale, J. K., Straus, S. E., & Hallett, M. (1996). Decreased postexercise facilitation of motor evoked potentials in patients with chronic fatigue syndrome or depression. *Neurology, 47,* 1410–1414.

Saphier, D. (1994, October). *A role for interferon in the psychoneuroendocrinology of chronic fatigue syndrome.* Paper presented at the American Association of Chronic Fatigue Syndrome Research Conference, Ft. Lauderdale, FL.

Schaefer, K. M. (1995). Sleep disturbances and fatigue in woman with fibromyalgia and chronic fatigue syndrome. *Journal of Obstetric, Gynecologic & Neonatal Nursing, 24,* 229–233.

Schlaes, J. L., & Jason, L. A. (1996). A buddy/mentor program for people with Chronic Fatigue Syndrome. *The CFIDS Chronicle, 9,* 21–25.

Schluederberg, A., Straus, S. E., Peterson, P., Blumenthal, S., Komaroff, A. L., Spring, S. B., Landay, A., & Buchwald, D. (1992). Chronic Fatigue Syndrome research: Definition and medical outcome assessment. *Annals of Internal Medicine, 117,* 325–331.

Schmaling, K., & DiClementi, J. D. (1995). Interpersonal stressors in chronic fatigue syndrome: A pilot study. *Journal of Chronic Fatigue Syndrome, 1,* 153–158.

Schmaling, K. B., & Jones, J. F. (1996). MMPI profiles of patients with Chronic Fatigue Syndrome. *Journal of Psychosomatic Research, 40,* 67–74.

Schor, J. (1991). *The overworked American: The unexpected decline of leisure.* New York: Basic Books.

Schwartz, J. E., Jandorf, L., & Krupp, L. B. (1993). The measurement of fatigue: A new instrument. *Journal of Psychosomatic Research, 37,* 753–762.

See, D. M., & Tilles, J. G. (1996). Alpha interferon treatment of patients with Chronic Fatigue Syndrome. *Immunological Investigations, 25,* 153–164.

Seeman, T. E., Berkman, L. F., Blazer, D., & Rowe, J. W. (1994). Social ties and support and neuroendocrine function: The MacArthur studies of successful aging. *Annals of Behavioral Medicine, 16*, 95–106.

Shafran, S. D. (1991). The Chronic Fatigue Syndrome. *The American Journal of Medicine, 90*, 730–739.

Shanks, M. F., & Ho-Yen, D. O. (1995). A clinical study of Chronic Fatigue Syndrome. *British Journal of Psychiatry, 166*, 798–801.

Sharpe, M. (1996, October). *Cognitive behavioral therapy: Implications for CFS.* Paper presented at the research conference of the American Association for Chronic Fatigue Syndrome, San Francisco.

Sharpe, M. C., Archard, L. C., Banatvala, J. E., Borysiewicz, L. K., Clare, A. W., David, A., Edwards, R. H. T., Hawton, K. E. H., Lambert, H. P., Lane, R. J. M., McDonald, E. M., Mowbray, J. F., Pearson, D. J., Peto, T. E. A., Preedy, V. R., Smith, A. P., Smith, D. G., Taylor, D. J., Tyrrell, D. A. J., Wessely, S., White, P. D., Behan, P. O., Rose, F. C., Peters, T. J., Wallace, P. G., Warrell, D. A., & Wright, D. J. M. (1991). A report-chronic fatigue syndrome: Guidelines for research. *Journal of the Royal Society of Medicine, 84*, 118–121.

Sharpe, M., Hawton, K., Simkin, S., Surawy, C., Hackmann, A., Klimes, I., Peto, T., Warrell, D., & Seagroatt, V. (1996). Cognitive behaviour therapy for the chronic fatigue syndrome: A randomised controlled trial. *British Medical Journal, 312*, 22–26.

Shorter, E. (1995). Sucker-punched again! Physicians meet the disease-of-the-month syndrome [Editorial]. *Journal of Psychosomatic Research, 39*, 115–118.

Siegel, B. (1986). *Love, medicine and miracles.* New York: Harper & Row.

Sigal, L. H. (1994). Persisting complaints attributed to chronic Lyme disease: Possible mechanisms and implications for management. *American Journal of Medicine, 96*, 365–374.

Silverstone, P. H. (1994). Poor efficacy of the Hospital Anxiety and Depression Scale in the diagnosis of major depressive disorder in both medical and psychiatric patients. *Journal of Psychosomatic Research, 38*, 441–450.

Smets, E. M. A., Garssen, B., Bonke, B., & de Haes, J. C. J. M. (1995). The multidimensional fatigue inventory (MFI): Psychometric qualities of an instrument to assess fatigue. *Journal of Psychosomatic Research, 39*, 315–325.

Smets, E. M. A., Garssen, B., Cull, A., & de Haes, J. C. J. M. (1996). Application of the multidimensional fatigue inventory (MFI-20) in cancer patients receiving radio therapy. *British Journal of Cancer, 73*, 241–245.

Snorrason, E., Geirsson, A., & Stefansson, K. (1996). Trial of selective acetylcholinesterase inhibitor, galanthamine hydrobromide, in the treatment of Chronic Fatigue Syndrome. *Journal of Chronic Fatigue Syndrome, 2*, 35–54.

Solomon, G. F., Temoshok, L., O'Leary, A., & Zich, J. (1987). An intensive psychoimmunologic study of long-surviving persons with AIDS. *Annals of the New York Academy of Sciences, 496*, 647–655.

Spacapan, S., & Oskamp, S. (1992). *Helping and being helped.* Newbury Park, CA: Sage.

Steele, L., Dobbins, J. G., Fukuda, K., Reyes, M., Randall, B., Koppelman, M., & Reeves, W. C. (in press). The epidemiology of chronic fatigue in San Francisco. *American Journal of Medicine.*

Steele, L., Reyes, M., & Dobbins, J. (1994, October). *The clinical course of Chronic Fatigue Syndrome (CFS): Longitudinal observation of CDC surveillance system participants.* Paper presented at the American Association of Chronic Fatigue Syndrome Research Conference, Ft. Lauderdale, FL.

Stewart, A. L., Hays, R. D., & Ware, J. E. (1988). The MOS Short-Form General Health Survey. Reliability and validity in a patient population. *Medical Care, 26*, 724–735.

Stone, A. A., Broderick, J. E., Porter, L. S., Krupp, L., Gnys, M., Paty, J. A., & Shiffman, S. (1994). Fatigue and mood in Chronic Fatigue Syndrome patients: Results of a momentary assessment protocol examining fatigue and mood levels and diurnal patterns. *Annals of Behavioral Medicine, 16,* 228–234.

Straus, S. (1992). Defining the Chronic Fatigue Syndrome. *Archives of Internal Medicine, 152,* 1559–1570.

Straus, S. E., Dale, J. K., Tobi, M., Lawley, T., & Preble, O. (1988). Acyclovir treatment of the chronic fatigue syndrome. Lack of efficiency in a placebo-controlled trial. *New England Journal of Medicine, 26,* 1692–1698.

Straus, S. E., Dale, J. K., Wright, R., & Metcalfe, D. D. (1988). Allergy and the chronic fatigue syndrome. *Journal of Allergy and Clinical Immunology, 81,* 791–795.

Straus, S. E., Fritz, S., Dale, J. K., Gould, B., & Strober, W. (1993). Lymphocyte phenotype and function in the Chronic Fatigue Syndrome. *Journal of Clinical Immunology, 13,* 30–40.

Strayer, D. R., Carter, W. A., Brodsky, I., Cheney, P., Peterson, D., Salvato, P., Thompson, C., Loveless, M., Shapiro, D. E., Elsasser, W., & Gillespie, D. H. (1994). A controlled clinical trial with a specifically configured RNA drug, poly(I)poly (C$_{12}$U), in Chronic Fatigue Syndrome. *Clinical Infectious Diseases, 18*(Suppl. 1), S88–S95.

Strayer, D. R., Carter, W. A., Strauss, K. I., Brodsky, I., & Suhadolnik, R. J. (1995). Long term improvements in patients with chronic fatigue syndrome treated with Ampligen. *Journal of Chronic Fatigue Syndrome, 1,* 35–53.

Stricklin, A., Sewell, M., & Austad, C. (1990). Objective measurement of personality variables in epidemic neuromyasthenia patients. *South African Medical Journal, 77,* 31–34.

Surawy, C., Hackmann, A., Hawton, K., & Sharpe, M. (1995). Chronic fatigue syndrome: A cognitive approach. *Behavior Research and Therapy, 33,* 535–544.

Swan, L. (1996). Occupational therapy: A new approach for persons with CFS. *The CFIDS Chronicle, Spring,* 48–49.

Tack, B. (1990a). A measure of fatigue in rheumatoid arthritis. *Arthritis Care and Research, 3,* 153.

Tack, B. (1990b). Self-reported fatigue in rheumatoid arthritis: A pilot study. *Arthritis Care and Research, 3,* 154–157.

Taerk, G. S., Toner, B. B., Salit, I. E., Garfinkel, P. E., & Ozersky, S. (1987). Depression in patients with neuromyasthenia (Benign Myalgic Encephalomyelitis). *International Journal of Psychiatry in Medicine, 17,* 49–56.

Taylor, R., & Jason, L. A., (in press). Psychiatric comorbidity and Chronic Fatigue Syndrome. *Psychology and Health: The International Review of Health Psychology.*

Thase, M. F. (1991). Assessment of depression in patients with chronic fatigue syndrome. *Reviews of Infectious Diseases, 13*(Suppl.), S114–S118.

Thoits, P. A. (1995). Stress, coping, and social support processes: Where are we? What next? [Special Issue]. *Journal of Health & Social Behavior,* 53–79.

Thomas, P. D., Goodwin, J. M., & Goodwin, J. S. (1985). Effects of social support on stress-related changes in cholesterol level, uric acid and immune function in an elderly sample. *American Journal of Psychiatry, 142,* 735–737.

Tiersky, L. A., Johnson, S. K., Lange, G., Natelson, B. H., & DeLuca, J. (1997). Neuropsychology of chronic fatigue syndrome. A critical review. *Journal of Clinical & Experimental Neuropsychology, 19,* 560–586.

Tollison, C. D., & Hinnant, D. W. (1996). Psychological testing in the evaluation of the patient in pain. In N. S. Waldman and A. P. Winnie (Eds.), *Interventional pain management* (pp. 119–128). Philadelphia: W. B. Saunders.

Trigwell, P., Hatcher, S., Johnson, M., Stanley, P., & Honse, A. (1995). "Abnormal" illness behavior in chronic fatigue syndrome and multiple sclerosis. *British Medical Journal, 311,* 15–18.

Trijsburg, R. W., Van Knippenberg, F. C., & Rijpma, S. E. (1992). Effects of psychological treatment on cancer patients: A clinical review. *Psychosomatic Medicine, 54,* 489–517.

Tryon, W. W. (1991). *Activity measurement in psychology and medicine* (pp. 23–63). New York: Plenum.

Tryon, W. W., & Williams, R. (1996). Fully proportional actigraphy: A new instrument. *Behavior Research Methods, Instruments, & Computers, 28,* 392–403.

Tubesing, N. L., & Tubesing, D. A. (1983). Getting out of my box. In N. L. Tubesing & D. A. Tubesing (Eds.), *Structured exercises in stress management* (pp. 89–99). Duluth, MN: Whole Person Press.

Turk, D. C., Meichenbaum, D., & Genest, M. (1983). *Pain and behavioral medicine.* New York: Guilford Press.

Turk, D. C., & Okifuji, A. (1994). Detecting depression in chronic pain patients: Adequacy of self reports. *Behavior Research and Therapy, 32,* 9–16.

Turk, D. C., & Rudy, T. E. (1988). Toward an empirically derived taxonomy of chronic pain patients: Integration of psychological assessment data. *Journal of Consulting and Clinical Psychology, 56,* 233–238.

Turk, D. C., & Rudy, T. E. (1990). The robustness of an empirically derived taxonomy of chronic pain patients. *Pain, 43,* 27–35.

Twemlow, S. W., Bradshaw, S. L., Jr., Coyne, L., Lerma, B. H. (1995). Some interpersonal and attitudinal factors characterizing patients satisfied with

medical care. *Psychological Reports, 77,* 51–59.

Twemlow, S. W., Bradshaw, S. L., Jr., Coyne, L., & Lerma, B. H. (1997). Patterns of utilization of medical care and perceptions of the relationship between doctor and patient with chronic illness including chronic fatigue syndrome. *Psychological Reports, 80,* 643–659.

Van Houdenhove, B., Onghena, P., Neerinckx, E., & Hellin, J. (1995). Does high "action-proneness" make people more vulnerable to Chronic Fatigue Syndrome? A controlled psychometric study. *Journal of Psychosomatic Research, 39,* 633–640.

Vercoulen, J. H. M. M., Swanink, C. M. A., Fennis, J. F. M., Galama, J. M. D., van der Meer, J. W. M., & Bleijenberg, G. (1996). Prognosis in chronic fatigue syndrome: A prospective study on the natural course. *Journal of Neurology, Neurosurgery, and Psychiatry, 60,* 489–494.

Vercoulen, J. H. M. M., Swanink, C. M. A., Zitman, F. G., Vreden, G. S., & Hoofs, M. P. E. (1996). Randomized, double-blind, placebo-controlled study of fluoxetine in chronic fatigue syndrome. *The Lancet, 347,* 858–862.

Vollmer-Conna, U., Hickie, I., Hadzi-Pavlovic, D., Tymms, K., Wakefield, D., Dwyer, J., & Lloyd, A. (1997). Intravenous immunoglobulin is ineffective in the treatment of chronic fatigue syndrome. *American Journal of Medicine, 103,* 38–43.

Wachtel, T., Piette, J., & Mor, V. (1992). Quality of life in persons with AIDS, as measured by the Medical Outcome Study's instruments. *Annals of Internal Medicine, 116,* 129–137.

Wallston, K. A. (1989). Assessment of control and healthcare settings. In A. Steptoe & A. Appels (Eds.), *Stress, personal control and health* (pp. 85–106). New York: Wiley.

Wallston, K. A. (1992). Hocus-pocus, the focus isn't strictly on locus: Rotter's social learning theory modified for health. *Cognitive Therapy and Research, 16*, 183–199.

Ware, J. E., Johnston, S. A., Davies-Avery, A. (1979). *Conceptualization and measurement of health for adults in the health insurance study: Vol. III: mental health* (Publication No. R-1987/3-HEW). Santa Monica, CA: Rand Corporation.

Ware, J. E., & Sherbourne, C. D. (1992). The MOS 36-item Short-Form Health Survey (SF-36): Conceptual framework and item selection. *Medical Care, June*, 473–483.

Ware, N. C. (1993). Society, mind and body in chronic fatigue syndrome: An anthropological view. In G. R. Boch & J. Whelan (Eds.), *Chronic fatigue syndrome* (pp. 62–81). New York: Wiley.

Ware, N. C., & Kleinman, A. (1992). Culture and somatic experience: The social course of illness in Neurasthenia and Chronic Fatigue Syndrome. *Psychosomatic Medicine, 54*, 546–560.

Wassem, R. (1991). A test of the relationship between health locus of control and the course of multiple sclerosis. *Rehabilitation Nursing, 16*, 189–193.

Watson, D., & Pennebaker, J. W. (1989). Health complaints, stress and distress: Exploring the central role of negative affectivity. *Psychological Review, 96*, 233–254.

Waylonis, G. W., & Perkins, R. H. (1994). Post-traumatic fibromyalgia: A long-term follow-up. *American Journal of Physical Medicine & Rehabilitation, 73*, 403–412.

Wearden, A., & Appleby, L. (1997). Cognitive performance and complaints of cognitive impairment in chronic fatigue syndrome (CFS). *Psychological Medicine, 27*, 81–90.

Wessely, S. (1990). Old wine in new bottles: Neurasthenia and "ME." *Psychological Medicine, 20*, 35–53.

Wessely, S. (1993). The neuropsychiatry of chronic fatigue syndrome. In B. R. Bock & J. Whelan (Eds.), *Chronic Fatigue Syndrome* (pp. 212–229). New York: Wiley.

Wessely, S. (1996, March). *Chronic fatigue syndrome*. Paper presented at the fourth International Congress of Behavioral Medicine, Washington, DC.

Wessely, S., Chalder, T., Hirsch, S., Pawlikowska, T., Wallace, P., & Wright, D. J. M. (1995). Postinfectious fatigue: Prospective cohort study in primary care. *The Lancet, 345*, 1333–1338.

Wessely, S., Chalder, T., Hirsch, S., Wallace, P., & Wright, D. (1997). The prevalence and morbidity of chronic fatigue and chronic fatigue syndrome: A prospective primary care study. *American Journal of Public Health, 87*, 1449–1455.

Wessely, S., & Powell, R. (1989). Fatigue syndromes: A comparison of chronic postviral fatigue with neuromuscular and affective disorders. *Journal of Neurology, Neurosurgery and Psychiatry, 52*, 940–948.

Westbrook, M. T., Gething, L., & Bradbury B. (1987). Belief in ability to control chronic illness: Associated evaluations and medical experiences. *Australian Psychologist, 22*, 203–218.

Whelton, C. L., Salit, I., & Moldofsky, H. (1992). Sleep, Epstein-Barr virus infection, musculoskeletal pain, and depressive symptoms in Chronic Fatigue Syndrome. *The Journal of Rheumatology, 19*, 939–943.

White, K. P., & Nielson, W. R. (1995). Cognitive–behavioral treatment of fibromyalgia: A follow-up assessment. *Journal of Rheumatology, 22*, 717–721.

White, P. D., & Cleary, K. J. (1997). An open study of the efficacy and adverse effects of moclobemide in patients with the chronic fatigue syndrome. *International Clinical Psychopharmacology, 12*, 47–52.

Willcockson, N. K. (1985). Discrimination of brain-damaged from functional psychiatric and medical patients with the MMPI. *Proceedings of the 1985 clinical psychology short course*, Letterman Army Medical Center, Presidio of San Francisco.

Williams, G., Pirmohamed, J., Minors, D., Waterhouse, J., Buchan, I., Arendt, J., & Edwards, R. H. T. (1996). Dissociation of body-temperature and melatonin secretion circadian rhythms in patients with Chronic Fatigue Syndrome. *Clinical Physiology, 16*, 327–337.

Wilson, A., Hickie, I., Lloyd, A., Hadzi-Pavlovic, D., Boughton, C., Dwyer, J., & Wakefield, D. (1994). Longitudinal study of outcome of chronic fatigue syndrome. *British Medical Journal, 308*, 756–759.

Wolfe, F., Smythe, H. A., Yunus, M. B., Bennett, R. M., & Bombardier, C. (1990). The American College of Rheumatology 1990 criteria for the classification of fibromyalgia. *Arthritis and Rheumatism, 33*, 160–172.

Wood, C., Magnello, M. E., & Sharpe, M. C. (1992). Fluctuations in perceived energy and mood among patients with chronic fatigue syndrome. *Journal of the Royal Society of Medicine, 85*, 195–198.

Wood, G. C., Bentall, R. P., Gopfert, M., Dewey, M. E., & Edwards, R. H. T. (1994). The differential response of chronic fatigue, neurotic and muscular dystrophy patients to experimental psychological stress. *Psychological Medicine, 24*, 357–364.

Woodward, R. V., Broom, D. H., & Legge, D. G. (1995). Diagnoses in chronic illness: Disabling or enabling—the case of chronic fatigue syndrome. *Journal of the Royal Society of Medicine, 88*, 325–329.

Wu, A. W., Rubin, H. R., Matthews, W. C., Ware, J. E., Jr., Brysk, L. T., Hardy, W. D., & Bozette, L. (1991). A health status questionnaire using 30 items from the medical outcomes study: Preliminary validation in persons with early HIV infection. *Medical Care, 29*, 786–798.

Yatham, L. N., Morehouse, R. L., Chisholm, B. T., Haase, D. A., MacDonald, D., & Marrie, J. J. (1995). Neuroendocrine assessment of serotonin (5-HT) function in chronic fatigue syndrome. *Canadian Journal of Psychiatry, 40*, 93–96.

Younger, J., Marsh, K. J., & Grap, M. J. (1995). The relationship of health, locus of control and cardiac rehabilitation to mastery of illness related stress. *Journal of Advanced Nursing, 22*, 294–299.

Zigmond, A. S., & Snaith, R. P. (1983). The Hospital Anxiety and Depression Scale. *Acta Psychiatrica Scandinavia, 67*, 361–370.

Zivin, J. A., & Choi, D. W. (1991). Stroke therapy. *Scientific American, 265*, 56–63.

Zung, W. W. K. (1965). A self-rating depression scale. *Archives of General Psychiatry, 12*, 63–70.

Author Index

Subject Index

About the Authors

Fred Friedberg, PhD, is clinical assistant professor of psychiatry in the Department of Psychiatry and Behavioral Sciences at the State University of New York at Stony Brook. He also maintains a private practice in Stony Brook, New York and New Milford, Connecticut. Friedberg has authored the popular book *Chronic Fatigue Syndrome: Nine Things You Can Do* (1995) and coauthored the professional volume *Hypnotherapy: A Modern Approach* (1987). He has also written articles that have appeared in *American Psychologist, Professional Psychology: Research and Practice, Journal of Cognitive Psychotherapy, Archives of Neurology, Clinical Infectious Diseases, Journal of Neuropsychiatry and Clinical Neurosciences,* and the *Journal of Chronic Fatigue Syndrome.* Friedberg has served on grant review committees for chronic fatigue syndrome (CFS) and HIV/AIDS for the National Institutes of Health (NIH). His clinical and research interests focus on CFS, chronic pain, and Eye Movement Desensitization and Reprocessing (EMDR). His most recent book, *Do It Yourself Eye Movement Therapy,* will be published in 1999.

Leonard A. Jason, PhD, is a professor of psychology at DePaul University. He received his PhD in clinical and community psychology from the University of Rochester. Jason is a former president of the Division of Community Psychology of the American Psychological Association (APA) and a past editor of *The Community Psychologist.* He received the 1997 Distinguished Contributions to Theory and Research Award from the Society for Community Research and Action (Division 27 of the APA). Jason has published more than 320 articles and chapters on preventive school-based interventions; the prevention of alcohol, tobacco, and other drug abuse; media interventions; program evaluation; and CFS. He has served on the editorial boards of 10 psychological journals and has edited or written 11 books. His most recent book is titled *Remote Control: A Sensible Guide for Kids, TV, and the New Electronic Media* (1997). Jason has served on review committees of the National Institute of Drug Abuse and the National Institute of

Mental Health and has received more than $6.35 million in federal research grants. He has received three media awards from the APA and is frequently asked to comment on policy issues for numerous media outlets.

In 1995, Jason was awarded a grant from NIH to study the epidemiology of CFS. Finally, he was presented the 1997 CSN ACTION Champion Award by the Chronic Fatigue Immune Dysfunction Syndrome Association of America in appreciation of research and educational efforts in behalf of persons with CFS.